# THE
# PRAYER
# DIET

# THE PRAYER DIET

*The Unique Physical, Mental and Spiritual Approach to Healthy Weight Loss*

## Matthew Anderson, D.Min.

CITADEL PRESS
Kensington Publishing Corp.
www.kensingtonbooks.com

CITADEL PRESS books are published by

Kensington Publishing Corp.
850 Third Avenue
New York, NY 10022

All Kensington titles, imprints, and distributed lines are available at
special quantity discounts for bulk purchases for sales promotions,
premiums, fund-raising, educational, or institutional use. Special
book excerpts or customized printings can also be created to fit
specific needs. For details, write or phone the office of the
Kensington special sales manager: Kensington Publishing Corp.,
850 Third Avenue, New York, NY 10022, attn: Special Sales
Department, phone 1-800-221-2647.

First Citadel printing: September 2001
First paperback printing: January 2004

10   9   8   7   6   5   4   3   2   1

Printed in the United States of America

Library of Congress Control Number: 2001091728

ISBN 0-8065-2612-2

To Jolynn, my dearest love and my partner through it all.

Every writer knows that many people contribute to the creation and publication of a book. I would like to say an enthusiastic "thank you" to some of them.

To Claire Gerus who envisioned the project and had the courage and perseverance to make it a reality.

To my wife, Jolynn, who has always been my most passionate encourager, supporter and perceptive editor.

To my eDiets.com editor, John McGran, who introduced me to the world of the Internet and then became one of my dearest colleagues.

To Mom and Dad who always remembered me in their prayers.

To Coleman Barks and Daniel Ladinsky whose respective translations of Rumi and Hafiz have taken me to new and amazing levels in my spiritual development.

To the Master of my heart who never ceases to love and challenge me more than I think I can imagine.

Matthew Anderson     June, 2001     Boca Raton, Florida

# Contents

———— ⌗ ————

# INTRODUCTION

*Start a huge, foolish, project,*
*like Noah.*
*It makes absolutely no difference*
*what people think of you.*

—Jelaludin Rumi


This book and the Dieter's Prayer exist as a result of a prayer, a dream, a lesson and a second prayer.

The first prayer brought a dream that gave me a vision for the second half of my life. The dream also introduced me to the most important spiritual lesson I have ever encountered. The second prayer has been answered so powerfully that it has dramatically changed my body—I lost over fifty pounds in six months—my work and my relationship with God.

When my fiftieth birthday arrived, I developed a growing concern: Was this the way it was going to be? Had I reached my final plateau? Was my current level of work and self-actualization going to be "it"? Was the rest of my life set, defined and limited by my present circumstances?

And yet, my life, by any standard, was good. My marriage was happy, my children were healthy, my counseling practice was busy and my health was fine, except that I was overweight. But I had a growing sense of fear that this was as good as it gets—and that was not good enough. Something was missing, and that something became more and more important as my fiftieth year progressed. Then, I began to pray about it.

For me, prayer is an intense, personal and intimate experience. I don't take it lightly. I talk to God just the way I talk to my wife, and his reactions are often similar. The prayer went like this:

"I need direction. I'm getting very upset about my life. I am becoming afraid that this is as good as it gets, and I don't like that. Help me out. Tell me it's going to change for the better. Give me some guidance. Send me a message in a dream. Please."

Why did I ask for a dream? Because dreams have always been major sources of healing and life direction for me. I keep dream journals and I have spent significant time in Jungian analysis learning about the transformative power of dreams. I also believe that God speaks to us in dreams. I could not think of a more appropriate request than "Send me a dream." So I prayed every night for a dream that would direct my life. Nothing happened.

I was so upset and impatient that I wrote the following in my dream journal: "I have been afraid for months that 'this' is all I will ever do or be—that my best gifts will be barely used and my life will not be a lesson learned and then shared, but will end in quiet mediocrity."

Two weeks had passed, and I had not remembered a

single dream. I became increasingly frustrated, but I also thought I knew what was happening. God was saying, "Relax. Give up the tension. Everything will occur in my time, not yours." I have been aware of this spiritual reality and divine characteristic since I was a little boy but never liked it. I wanted the dream now. I was frustrated, and I continued to pray. On about the fifteenth night I had a dream.

The dream had such a significant effect on my life that I still get tears in my eyes when I reflect upon it. It occurred on July 19, 1996:

> *I am reading a book of sacred sayings. I look at the left-hand column of the left page, the second saying from the top. I intuitively know it is just for me—a message. It is only four lines long. As I read, I have a visual image of being halfway across a Japanese-style bridge:*

> *You are only halfway across the bridge.*
> *Don't define yourself by halfway.*
> *You are not finished.*
> *You will be O.K.*

> *I am filled with an overwhelming awareness that I have much more to do and accomplish. I feel enormously relieved that I am not "over." I begin to sob with joy and relief.*

I woke up sobbing. My prayer had been answered with incredible grace. God had responded with more clarity and specificity than I had hoped for. I was touched and satisfied and cried some more.

A few weeks later, I decided I was supposed to write a book. I made an outline and began to write. That is when I was taught the lesson contained in the dream. It was in the image of the bridge.

I was sitting on the couch in my office writing the title to a chapter in the book. I wrote the words "Commitment and Surrender." I looked at the title and decided I was only going to write about commitment. It was a subject I felt I knew a lot about and had great enthusiasm for. I scratched out "Surrender" and proceeded to forget about it.

Ten minutes passed, and my essay on commitment was flowing nicely. There was a knock at the door, and my friend and colleague Santo appeared. Santo is a Jungian analyst who had an office next to mine. He asked me what I was doing, and we began to chat about my book, his travels and the Florida heat.

In the midst of our conversation I had a strong urge to tell Santo about my dream. We often shared dreams and explored their interpretations. I have always appreciated his perceptive insights and had an intuition that I needed his feedback on this particular dream.

When I finished describing the dream, Santo had an observation and a question that stunned me. He said that Carl Jung often talked about bridges, especially bridges that symbolized being halfway finished with life. Dr. Jung used to say that people in my position need to consider one thing: What worked in the first half of life will not work in the second half. Santo looked at me and asked if that brought anything to mind.

I was stunned. I immediately knew the answer and the lesson. The first half of my life, I had been a rebel. I called it "being independent", "being my own person", "doing my own thing." Rebellion had been a central part of my personality and lifestyle. I had always refused to surrender, and I directed my own goals and future. Tony Robbins would have been proud.

Everyone has the ability to become immediately aware of inner truth. Sometimes it just appears and there is nothing we can do to deny it. For me, this was one of those moments. I had lived without surrender. Now I had to learn it. It was no surprise that I had just attempted to drop the word from the chapter I was writing. I had never experienced it.

Now I was flooded with childhood memories. I remembered being in church Sunday after Sunday and singing the hymn, "I Surrender All" at the end of the service. I knew every word and note but could never heed the hymn's words. Oh, I joined the church, gave my life to Jesus and even received a "call" to the ministry, but I never surrendered. Now the dream was telling me that I had no choice. It was time to learn a new lesson.

Over the next few years, I struggled with the idea of surrender and was confronted by a difficult reality. I could no longer control my life. I would set a goal, make plans and start productive action toward the goal's accomplishment. But nothing would happen. I would be frustrated and powerless. Then I would remember the lesson and let go. Surrender means trusting and not being in control. I discovered that every once in a while I could actually do it . . . let go and trust.

Sometimes events occurred that made me feel happy and productive, but overall I remained frustrated. I was trying to surrender, but my work life remained mediocre. I was plagued by a recurring mental image. I imagined I was an enormous warehouse full of large, unopened boxes. Each box contained items that were extremely valuable but were undiscovered. Hundreds of people would enter the warehouse, but never ventured past the small entry room. I was unable to get anyone to explore the hidden wealth right under their noses. I felt powerless, helpless and totally at the mercy of God's divine will.

I constantly reminded myself that the dream was authentic and that I needed to surrender before anything could happen. I did not like the process, but I was clearly aware that I was not in charge. Finally, I began to pray the second prayer.

The second prayer went like this:

*"I need your help again. I am so frustrated I could pop my cork. I have a warehouse full of valuable stuff I am dying to share, and nobody seems to want it. Please use me. Don't let me go to waste. Use everything I've got for your purposes. I know I can't make any of this happen under my own power. I know I can't direct my own life. I give up. I surrender. Please use me for all I'm worth. Thy will be done."*

I wasn't kidding, and I think God knew it. I was finally ready. Then I got a call from eDiets.

Actually, the call came from my friend John McGran, who had just become managing editor for the newly-blossoming diet resource dot-com called eDiets.com. John asked me if I would like to write an article for the newsletter. I immediately said yes and we discussed the topic. Instead of weight loss, we agreed that the article would be about guidelines for handling and surviving extreme stress. I had led a recent workshop on the subject and had lots of material ready.

I told John the material would require my writing five articles instead of only the one he had proposed. He did some thinking and agreed to two articles, with the proviso that three more would follow if the eDiets readers responded. In February 2000, my first article was published. Both articles received enthusiastic responses from readers, and by the end of week five, eDiets had asked me to begin a weekly column.

If there is a secret to having a prayer answered, it is contained in this experience. When John called me, I had owned a computer for only one year. I went on-line for about an hour per week and that was to play games or read the few e-mails I received. I had no idea how to send even the simplest attachment, much less forward an article to eDiets. For the first six or eight weeks, I put my articles on disk and drove them to John's office. By the grace of God, the eDiets headquarters was only five minutes from my home.

The secret to answered prayer is openness. Once we pray a prayer, we must allow ourselves to become completely open to an answer that might not meet our expectations. Otherwise, we might miss God's reply altogether, and that can be a tragedy.

I never expected to be an Internet columnist, and I never dreamed it would lead to the creation of a book about prayer and weight loss. But I am now used to God's sense of humor, so I said yes when the opportunity arrived.

My eDiets column, entitled "Coyote Wisdom," quickly became successful, and I was soon offered a contract to write two columns a week. In July 2000, I wrote the article called "The Prayer Diet." That article changed my life—and the lives of millions of others.

A normal weight-loss diet usually directs the dieter toward the best foods and away from the worst, or most fattening, foods. This weight-loss diet is not about food. Contrary to popular belief, food is not the real cause of weight gain. That's why diets that focus on food alone are doomed to fail. This diet is literally what it says it is—a diet of prayer. Instead of watching what you eat, this diet teaches you what to pray, how to pray and when to pray. Prayer will become your central source of sustenance, and its power will help you overcome the deeper causes of overeating and weight gain.

The Prayer Diet has a central and particular prayer as its focus. But that prayer is supported by a number of other prayers that will help you heal, change and transform your relationship to food, yourself and God. As you follow the simple guidelines of the Prayer Diet, you will find yourself more and more immersed in a life of natural and life-giving prayer that will help you lose weight. You will also discover that weight loss is only one of the wonderful gifts that will appear with a daily diet of prayer.

As you progress on your prayer and weight-loss journey, you may even begin to see your excess weight as God's mysterious and unpredictable way of drawing you closer to his love and care. It has certainly been that way for me and for many others who have participated in this program. I invite you, therefore, to begin the prayers today and to prepare yourself for an endless chain of miracles.

> *What if you could pray for anything you wanted and the answer was better than you could imagine? Where would you start?*

# THE
# PRAYER
# DIET

# One

# HOW I CAME TO PRAYER

——————— ∞ ———————

*"We can't help being thirsty,*
*moving toward the voice*
*of water.*

*Milk drinkers draw close*
*to the mother. Muslims, Christians, Jews,*
*Buddhists, Hindus, shamans,*
*Everyone hears the intelligent sound*
*and moves, with thirst, to meet it.*

*Clean your ears. Don't listen*
*for something you've heard before."*

—Jelaludin Rumi

——————— ∞ ———————

Icame to prayer the same way a fish comes to water. I was born into it.

South Carolina is as close to being the "buckle" of the Bible Belt as a state can be. For me, a child born into a devout Baptist family, it could easily have been named "the Prayer Belt." Everybody I knew prayed. Prayer was a daily fact, a reality and a ritual that threaded its way through the fabric of my everyday existence.

I remember the first prayer I was taught. I prayed it every night before I went to sleep. My mother taught it to me, and I always think fondly of her when I hear it.

*Now I lay me down to sleep. I pray the Lord my soul to keep. If I should die before I wake, I pray the Lord my soul to take. Amen.*

Some say this prayer is not good for children because it makes them afraid of the possibility of death. But it never frightened me. In fact, it made me feel good and safe. I liked the rhyme, and I liked the idea that the Lord would be there for me. I discovered much later in life that the practice of confronting death is common among Tibetan Buddhists who say we never know which world we will wake up in—this one or the next.

I believe the Tibetans have the right idea. Death is a reality of life. We cannot be fully alive until we are willing to live with the presence of death. Any prayer that helps us confront that truth is a good one.

As devout Baptists, we spent a lot of time in church. Sunday was church day, morning and evening, with lunch and a nap in between. Then, on Wednesday evening, we frequently attended prayer meeting. It was an hour of praying about everything and everyone, with a short message by the minister. Baptists cannot resist the urge to preach, but, thankfully, our pastor always kept it short.

Our family, like many "Belt" families, also prayed at every meal. I don't mean meals at home. I mean *every* meal, at home or in a restaurant. The prayer was usually given by the eldest male at the table, and my dad and grandfather had their own special prayers, which we always called "Blessings."

Dad's blessing went like this: *"Heavenly Father, make us thankful for these and all our blessings. In Christ's name, Amen."* Granddaddy's blessing was different: *"Blessed Father, forgive our sins and give us thankful hearts for these and all our blessings. In Christ's name, Amen."*

I heard these prayers thousands of times by the time I was twenty-one. They are imprinted on my heart and always bring an inner warmth and peace when I remember them.

The other prayer that dominated my childhood was the Lord's Prayer. Roman Catholics call this prayer the "Our Father," after the first two words. But I was in my late teens before I even knew a Catholic person. There was a small Catholic church across the street from our Baptist church but people of that religious persuasion were not part of my childhood. We prayed The Lord's Prayer at many church functions, but it remained a group ritual with little meaning for me until I was much older.

As a child, I often heard stories about the many miracles prayer could effect, and I believed them all. I had no reason not to. Everyone I knew and respected believed in the power of prayer, and everyone prayed. When I was twenty years old, I experienced my first prayer miracle.

I was a junior in college and deeply involved with a nineteen-year-old girl. We planned to marry the following year. One morning she called and said two words: "I'm late." My heart sank, and I couldn't breathe. I was young, but I was not stupid and I knew this was a catastrophe. "Late" meant pregnant, and pregnant meant big trouble for her and for me. My life passed quickly before my eyes.

Here I was, a good Christian boy on his way to seminary to become a minister. I had just been elected state president of the Baptist student union. I had a summer job scheduled as youth minister of a local Baptist church. I knew the news would devastate my mother, and my father would probably kill me. Life, as I knew it, was over. I would have to kiss college and the ministry good-bye, get a job at J.C. Penney's, marry my girlfriend and move into a trailer park.

I was in a panic. I had no idea what to do or who to talk to. For the next two weeks, I privately obsessed about the impending disaster, and I prayed what I now refer to as the classic "foxhole" prayer: *"Oh, God, please get me out of this one. Don't let her be pregnant, God. Please, please, please. Just let me out of this, and I promise I will never have sex until we are married."*

About fourteen painful days after the first call, I received another. "Hi, I just called to tell you that I got my period today." I fell to my knees. *"Thank you, thank you, thank you. Thank you for a miracle. Thank you for giving me my life back."*

I don't have proof my girlfriend was pregnant. She never took a test or saw a doctor. But to this day I believe I received a miracle as an answer to prayer. I have come to understand that miracles don't always arrive with total scientific confirmation. I think this leaves a little space for faith. So I was and am very grateful to God for His compassionate act. It is also clear that I still had a lot to learn about prayer.

I choose to share this unpleasant and humiliating experience because I want to make a very important point about prayer. This book is about prayer and weight loss. Many people feel that weight loss is too insignificant an issue for prayer. They also feel that being overweight is bad, or sinful, or indicative of character flaws. But prayer is for everyone, regardless of one's infirmities, problems or shortcomings. In fact, prayer is especially for these people.

I came to meaningful prayer in the midst of what I considered a life crisis. At that moment, I was more open and available than ever for communication with God. This kind of prayer is natural and easy. It seems to emerge from the soul and go straight to God's ear. It is a painful, but intimate, cry to the source of our existence that arises intuitively from our most human core.

I believe prayer is a natural act—it does not have to be learned. It is as normal as breathing. We can control it, and it occurs spontaneously when we need it. This is why many of us experience authentic prayer for the first time in the midst of a crisis. It is an involuntary reaction to our deepest need.

Was this pregnancy crisis placed in my path to teach me about prayer? I believe it was. Prayer was such an ordinary part of my everyday existence that I had no real appreciation of it. It was a ritual, but had not become a cry from my heart. It took a "wake-up" phone call to cause that.

My life has not been simple or easy. My most important lessons have been hard earned. I have fallen, jumped or been thrown into many potholes on the road of life. The pregnancy scare was comparatively low on the scale. But in the midst of my confusion, I learned about the life-giving, miracle-producing power of prayer. I exist, live and prosper because of it, and the God it has introduced me to.

Another reason I told the above story was to make this point: *Prayer is not for the pure.* Many people don't pray because they think they are not good enough to speak to God. They are under the mistaken impression that God requires us to be "happy, clean and pure" before we are allowed to enter his presence. Nothing could be more inaccurate.

No one is pure. Everyone makes mistakes and has come short of the glory of God. Everyone has their messes, their imperfections and their nasty selves. We are all mysterious mixtures of joyous light and disappointing darkness. No one is an exception. Therefore we need prayer. We cannot be without it.

Prayer is a wonderful antidote to our confusing

predicament. It provides us with a relationship with a Power that understands the mysterious human condition. It is a way out, a healing that puts the pieces of the puzzle together. It is our half of a relationship that brings us to the very essence of our humanity and our divinity. When we pray, God responds with more compassion, understanding and love than we can imagine, causing miracles to occur.

So God provided a miracle and said, "Go and sin no more." I was good for a while, then I went back to my old habits and finally we got married with no complications.

## Is There a Right Way To Pray?

Is there a special formula or order of words that God expects or demands? Growing up as a Christian, I initially believed that the Lord's Prayer was the be-all and end-all of prayer perfection. The prayer is beautiful. It has a simplicity and wholeness that has kept it at the center of Christian prayer for twenty centuries. But I do not believe that Jesus meant it to be an icon for the believer. He was too focused on the essential spirit of things to make the wording of the prayer a law. I think he would have loved the following story about prayer.

First, some background. Jelaludin Rumi is one of the world's most well-read and revered spiritual poets. He lived in Konya, Turkey, in the thirteenth century. Even though he was a Sufi, he has been studied and is deeply respected by spiritual seekers of all faiths. Rumi was a man who was passionately in love with God. His spiritual insights are a testimony to that love and its transforming effects on his life and work.

Since the early 1990s, I have been a devoted and happy student of this man. Although I do not consider myself a Rumi expert, I love his work and have been substantially influenced by his knowledge of the Divine Lover.

In one of his thousands of poems, Rumi tells a story about Moses and prayer. Since Rumi was a Muslim, this Moses was the same Moses mentioned in Jewish and Christian scripture. The story contains the essence of the true purpose and structure of prayer:

One day, Moses was walking through a village on an important journey for God. As he passed by a small house, he overheard a man praying. Moses was so shocked by what he heard he stopped and listened, aghast. "Oh, God, I love you so much I would do anything for you. Let me wash your little hands and little feet. Let me care for your every need."

Before the man could continue, Moses, in a fit of righteous anger, reached through the window and grabbed the man by his tunic. "Sir, what do you think you are doing? You cannot talk to God that way. God does not have little hands and feet. He does not need your care. Sir, you are blaspheming and you must stop now and never pray this way again."

The frightened man fell at Moses' feet, because he recognized the great spiritual leader. He begged for forgiveness and promised he would never again speak to

God in this fashion. Moses released the sinner and went on his way, still fuming at this inappropriate prayer.

Later that day, God came to Moses and spoke to him. "My son, what were you doing with my servant today? Why did you stop him from praying?"

Moses explained that the man was blaspheming and desperately needed instruction in the proper wording and attitude of prayer.

God became angry and said, "Moses, what have you done? You have made a serious mistake. Do you think I listen to the words that a man prays? No, I do not. I listen to the message of his heart. His heart is the bearer of his true prayer. You have done a grave injury to my devoted servant. Return to him and tell him his prayer was dear to me."

When Moses heard God's words, his heart was opened to the true meaning of prayer. He rushed to the village and found the man and told him God's message. From that day forth, Moses understood the essence of prayer—the attitude of the heart.

In prayer, words are not the issue, nor are they a requirement. God listens to the heart of one who prays; all else is window dressing.

Authentic prayer, prayer that touches God, is a matter of the heart and not of the vocabulary. Whether I pray for a sick friend, a child who is in pain, or my own weight loss, every true prayer goes from the heart straight to God's ear. Thank God.

## A Never-Ending Journey

Like a fish, I was born into a sea of prayer. And like a fish, I never really appreciated that sea and its life-giving function until I was snagged by the hook of a life crisis and deposited into a frightening emptiness. I assume that God was the compassionate fisherman who brought me to consciousness, then dropped me back into the ocean. From that moment, I had a new relationship with prayer.

My relationship with prayer is like any intimate relationship: always expanding and growing, yet remaining a mystery. Prayer is not a small book that is easily opened, read and understood. It is more like a huge library whose books cannot be consumed in one lifetime.

I began my journey to prayer as a child with a child's limited perception. As the years have passed, I have encountered many spiritual teachers who expanded my vision of this life-giving function. Each one broke down another wall that had obstructed my view and introduced me to greater nuances of this amazing mystery.

Jesus taught me, among other things, that God may be spoken to as "abba," a Hebrew word for an intimate version of "father." I will explore this in more depth later, but it essentially made God accessible and trustworthy to me. Professor Bedenbaugh, a New Testament teacher at a Lutheran Seminary I attended for a year, released me from my stilted, formalized wording and introduced me to direct, unselfconscious conversational prayer. Zen taught me that stillness and simplicity are both forms of prayer and prepared me to receive God's responses.

I have had many prayer teachers, and I constantly return to Jesus' guidance on the matter. But during the last ten years, Rumi has made a powerful contribution. He has made me aware of how praying can be a form of making love. God is my ultimate lover, and I am his beloved. Prayer is the vehicle that carries the passion.

I pray daily, and each day I learn a little more about prayer. I think the most useful lesson is that there is always more to learn. I knew that I could pray for others and for healing and guidance. I have prayed in the midst of life's trials and difficulties. I have recently learned, however, that I could pray for something as seemingly insignificant (I thought) as weight loss, and that has opened my eyes to a new level of prayer. It is the reason for this book.

# Two

# WEIGHT LOSS AS A PATH TO GOD

---

*Don't turn your head. Keep looking
at the bandaged place. That's where
the Light enters you.*

*And don't believe for a moment
that you're healing yourself.*

—Jelaludin Rumi

---

Many Americans are spiritually deprived. It is even more obvious that the majority of us are overweight and I believe there is a direct connection between the two. Now I want to make a third and even more important point: *Weight loss can be a path to God*.

Most of us have been taught to view excess weight as a problem. We see even the slightest obesity as ugly and unhealthy, and we flock to any program or technique that will remove it as quickly as possible. To us, fat is bad and we are bad for being fat. Fat has no purpose other than to remind us that we are indulgent overeaters. Period.

### Wounds Can Be Windows

I believe that fat hate is produced by minds and hearts that have not been introduced to the mysterious and purposeful works of God. If we remain stuck in and dominated by our society's myopic view of excess weight, we will miss one of God's most wonderful characteristics—the ability to use our wounds as windows.

Rumi invites us to look at the bandaged place *"Because that's where the light enters you."* Most of us experience our fat as a wound. Being fat hurts. It hurts our bodies, our relationships, our self-image and our self-esteem. Most of us hate being fat, and no one will get rich selling books that help us gain weight. To us, weight is certainly a wound and we are constantly in search of a healing solution.

In his wisdom, Rumi points us to a healing solution

that is paradoxical, yet potent. He is saying that we need to drop our normal way of looking at pain and begin to see it through "spiritual eyes." Spiritual vision almost always sees things opposite to the common view. It provides us with a transformational tool that helps us see light where we could only see darkness and suffering.

Initially, this type of vision requires courage. We have to do the very thing we would generally avoid—look at the bandaged place. We must stop, turn around and peer intently at the wound that we wish would disappear. We can no longer ignore the hurt and suffering the wound has caused us. And yet, Rumi and other spiritual teachers tell us that this is exactly what is necessary if we are to find its blessing.

Who among us can think of fat as a blessing? Most of us consider it a curse. But hating a wound never healed a wound, and our spiritual growth and ultimately, our weight loss depends on our willingness to see fat in a new way and thus discover its real and lasting blessing.

From 1981 to 1982 I was chaplain at the San Diego Hospice and visited patients who requested consultation with a minister. On one such visit, I met a seventy-year-old woman who had been told by her doctor that she had less than six months to live.

I was thirty-six years old and new to the chaplaincy, and assumed that this woman was unhappy about dying and wanted me to help her cope with this difficult passage. I was stunned to discover that I was wrong.

While trying to comfort her, I asked what had been the best year of her life. I naively believed this "perceptive inquiry" would direct her thoughts to more positive times. She smiled and gave me an answer I never anticipated.

> *"The best year of my life began the moment I was told that I had six months to live. Since that day, I have had a totally changed perspective on my life, my relationships and every single aspect of life itself. I have been able to let go of all the trivialities that always disturbed me. People don't annoy me anymore. I can see what's good in them and can tolerate the other less important stuff.*
>
> *I wake up every morning happy to greet whatever the weather brings. I love the sunshine and the rain and the clouds and the wind. I treasure every moment in a way that I was never able to experience it. I love being alive, and I love every happy and sad part of it.*
>
> *You may think I am crazy, but I am happy that I got cancer. Without it, I would never have lived."*

From the first sentence she uttered, I knew I was being given a gift and was able to keep quiet and take in her wisdom. In only a few moments, she had opened my inner vision. She had taken what most people would consider the worst news they could hear and transformed it into the best experience of her life.

The woman died within months of our conversation. I am sure she went peacefully. I remember her with a thankful heart because she taught me a lesson that has helped me confront and transform many of my own struggles: My wounds can become windows if I am willing to look with different eyes.

Since that special visit, I have met many other enlightened souls who have learned to see the Light in their wounds. These have included alcoholics and drug addicts, women with breast cancer, Holocaust survivors, victims of sexual and physical abuse, adults who have lost spouses, children and parents, and victims of almost every imaginable trauma or life crisis.

These individuals are not common and certainly are not in the majority, but they have found a gift that is worth all the suffering. They have learned to see life, not with their own eyes, but with God's eyes. When that is achieved, life holds no horrors.

If a seventy-year-old woman is able to change her experience with cancer from fear and loathing to wonder and love, shouldn't those of us who are obese be able to consider it in a different light? The process can begin with a prayer:

> *"I am stuck in fat-hate. I see being overweight as a wound. Please give me the vision to see the blessing contained in it. Please open my inner eyes and let me see your handiwork in this painful problem."*

---

*What if you came to see that your excess weight is actually a pathway that can lead you to the most wonderful gifts that God can give you? What would you pray for then?*

---

### Excess Weight: A Blessing in Disguise?

You and I have spent enough of our precious time hating fat. We have spent far too much time hating ourselves for being fat. Now it is time to change that perception and begin to see the gifts excess weight can lead us to. The first gift is the gift of faith.

> *"God's joy moves from unmarked box to unmarked box,*
> *from cell to cell. As rainwater, down into flowerbed.*
> *As roses up from ground.*
> *Now it looks like a plate of rice and fish,*
> *Now a cliff covered with vines,*
> *Now a horse being saddled.*
> *It hides within these,*
> *Till one day it cracks them open."*
>
> —Jelaludin Rumi

Faith grows best and helps best in the midst of difficulty. A life that is devoid of pain, confusion, hardship or abysses is a life that requires no faith. None of us has met a single soul who had led a life of total bliss and good fortune. We are all in need of the supportive and healing power that faith can provide.

I occasionally meet people who claim to have had no struggles in life. After closer inspection, I usually discover they are more victims of gross unconsciousness than lucky recipients of good fortune. In fact, no one is exempt from life's hardships and everyone can handle them better with the help of faith.

You are probably reading this book because you want to lose weight. You see your weight as a problem, and you want a solution. You probably also find the idea of praying for weight loss intriguing. You like the connection between spirituality and dieting. What do you imagine will happen to your faith if you pray and then lose weight? Will you trust in the power of prayer more than you did before you started? Will you pray more fervently about other areas of your life?

*Nothing helps our faith more than a problem that is resolved by an answer to prayer.* Faith tested is faith proved. If it is obvious to us, then it must be even more obvious to God. Why, then, would God hesitate to offer us opportunities to test and prove our faith? He would not hesitate. He constantly affords us myriad opportunities to open ourselves to his wisdom and care.

Am I saying that God makes us fat in order to help us grow our faith? I have asked myself and God this question a thousand times, and each time I receive an answer both complicated and paradoxical. It is a powerful question that goes far beyond the realm of weight loss. If God makes us fat to help us grow our faith, does he bring other sources of pain (such as disease, accidents, and loss) as well?

Every religion and serious spiritual seeker has grappled with this issue. Here is what I have come to believe.

God is far larger and more mysterious than any of us can imagine. Every time I construct a box for him to live in, he appears outside of it. If I think there is no way God can use or transform an experience in my life, I need only to wait. Something always emerges, and that something is always redemptive.

I cannot say whether or not God actually causes painful events to occur in order for us to grow. However, I can say that God is always capable of transforming our experience of these events. What initially appears to be a source of pain and despair can become a life-changing source of light, inspiration and healing. If that is always to be the case, and I have faith that it is, then I am willing to live happily with the mystery.


### Faith or Fear

> *"Fear is the cheapest room in the house.*
> *I would like to see you living*
> *In better conditions."*

> —Hafiz

Life's difficult events and passages offer us two choices: faith or fear. We can continue to be afraid of fat, cancer, accidents and loss or we can learn to have faith that these normal aspects of life can become agents of change, growth and healing.

I encounter many individuals who live from fear to fear. They are constantly beset by fears of illness, accident or attack. Freeways are full of accidents waiting to happen, foods are potential sources of toxins, parking lots are venues for robbery. Minor aches and pains are symptoms of greater disease, travel is an invitation to all three maladies (illness, accident or attack), relationships are almost guarantees of hurt and disappointment and authentic self-expression is a clear request for rejection.

It is rare that I meet someone without a few of these painful and life-constricting attitudes. The fear of life appears to be a growing disease that affects many of us, and it is particularly true of those who have chronic weight problems.

I have had the opportunity to explore these fears with many clients and workshop participants. I have also looked deeply into my own life terror. Two facts have emerged. One is that we have good reason to be afraid because we have all been hurt in one fashion or another. We learned to fear life because life caused us pain. We then generalized from the original discomfort to anything that may appear even vaguely similar. We are not crazy. We are simply trying to avoid being hurt again.

The second fact is this: *Not one single person I have met who has a major fear of life is a person of faith.* This is not a judgment on my part. It is a simple statement of fact. Faith and fear do not live well together. One moves the other out. If we allow fear to dominate us, it will color our perceptions of everything that arises in our lives.

I have presented the faith versus fear issue as if it is a choice because it is. But even if we have led a fear-dominated life, we can still have the ability to live a life centered in faith. Obviously, this shift is not an easy process. It takes effort and desire and a great deal of support.

In truth, we are already faithful. We are already skilled at trusting our lives to a power greater than ourselves. We who are frequently afraid are full of faith in our fear. We trust the messages our fear sends us over every other message we receive. We use our fear as a guide and a trusted friend. We go to it as if it can see deeply into the fabric of every situation that confronts us, and we even ascribe it with psychic, future-telling powers.

I often say to counselees that if they honor their fear more than their faith in God, they will live in terror and always feel the need to protect themselves from the worst.

The solution is to develop our faith in a loving, divine source that is always present and working through every aspect of our lives. We can accelerate this process of faith building by exploring God's lessons and gifts that are embedded in our weight issues.

I could not be more emphatic about this statement. Weight is an important life issue. You would not be reading this book if it were not. Given the reality of weight, why not allow it to become a source of something wonderful? Why not allow your weight struggle to be an agent of spiritual growth and let it move you into a deep and fearless experience of life itself?

## PRAYER: The First Step to Weight Loss

Let's assume you are very fat. For some, that means being twenty pounds overweight; for others it means 200 excess pounds. Whatever the number, you see yourself as fat and you hate it. You want to lose weight, and you want to keep it off. Nothing, however, has worked. You have tried many diet and exercise programs, and you have not been able to lose so much as a pound. Finally, in desperation, you turn to prayer.

For many of us, the decision to pray is a difficult one. We have never trusted it. Some of us even think of prayer as a child's pastime. We believe that adults are responsible for their own lives and are not supposed to ask God to help with something we should be taking care of ourselves. Praying would be a sign of weakness. We take pride in our independence, and prayer, any prayer, is an expression of dependence.

When I have asked independent personalities to describe the proper use of prayer, they usually have no answers. They are convinced that prayer is weakness and weakness is as bad or worse than being overweight.

Desperation, in the service of spiritual growth, can be a good thing. Many of us are like the people I have described. We believe we should be adults who are in charge of every aspect of our lives. This attitude is unrealistic and, in the extreme, dysfunctional, but we can't see it. Being desperate about our obesity may be the only crack in our defense against asking for help from God or anyone else.

So we try everything we can imagine, and we fail repeatedly. Then we give up and allow the true healing answers to appear.

*"Failure is the key
to the kingdom within.*

*Your prayer should be, 'Break the legs
of what I want to happen. Humiliate
my desire. Eat me like candy.
It's spring, and finally
I have no will.'"*

—Rumi

Rumi states a fact of spiritual reality. Failure marks the spot at which we learn to let go and let God do the work. For many of us, this is where we learn to truly pray for the first time in our lives.

We were desperate about losing weight. We tried everything. Finally, in defeat, we began to pray. It is no accident that this process sounds almost identical to the first step of Alcoholics Anonymous and every other twelve-step addiction program. Every recovering addict knows that real help cannot arrive until we admit we are powerless to control the addiction.

Being overweight is no different. Feeling powerless to lose weight, even if it is only five pounds, can bring us to a spiritual breakthrough that can change our weight and our entire existence. We begin to pray.

The act of prayer is not an act of weakness from a spiritual point of view. It is the beginning of real strength. Nothing could make us stronger than a direct connection to the source of all strength. What were we thinking? We had the whole thing backward and upside down. No wonder we could not change the size of our body. By refusing to pray, we were demonstrating our impotence, not our power. By deciding to pray, we have accessed the greatest power in the universe.

Finally we pray and then, miraculously, we begin to lose weight. Can it be true? Is this for real? Yes, the scale doesn't lie. We have lost two or five or fifty pounds. Our bodies are confirming the material and observable effects of prayer. What now?

Losing weight as a result of prayer may be the first time you have experienced a direct answer to prayer. It may shake your reality. Something out of the ordinary is occurring. What does it mean? What implications does it have for the rest of your life? What else should you pray for?

Any undeniable experience of the power of prayer can change a person's life. It can and will change yours. Something as ordinary and apparently mundane as weight loss can open you to an intimate relationship with God himself. Is this a good thing? Obviously. What should you do next? Keep praying!

### Excess Weight and the Gift of Surrender

Almost everything I said about prayer in the section above applies to the gift of surrender. Surrender is one of the greatest spiritual gifts a human being can experience. This truth is evident to devoted followers of all great religions. Total surrender to the will and direction of God is at the top of the spiritual mountain. Every devotee of every religious tradition must sooner or later come to terms with this frightening and liberating reality.

The prayer of surrender is, "Thy will be done." No other prayer is needed. At this point, the ego has been relinquished to divine will, and the obstructions to the flow of the divine in one's life are gone.

The journey to this transformational act is long and fraught with many difficulties, and we need all the help that God can give us to achieve it. I am convinced that the hardships of significant weight loss can help move us toward that goal.

For the last seven years, since I was fifty, I have struggled daily with the meaning of surrender in my journey to God. I have made some progress, though at times it seems to be minuscule, and I have had momentary visions of its real magnificence and incredible power of liberation. I am not an expert on the subject, but I can share a bit of what I have learned to help support your movement and growth.

Everyone who contemplates the idea of surrender is aware of the difficulties it brings. Surrender requires us to relinquish control of every aspect of our lives and submit ourselves to the loving direction of God. We can't do this easily because we have spent most of our existence trying to gain control and take charge of who and what we are. Surrender can seem like going backward or giving up in defeat.

Surrender also implies trust, which is not easy for any contemporary adult. We must learn to trust the divine source of love more than we trust our egos. To the ego, which has spent years growing, developing and directing our daily existence, this appears to be an invitation to suicide.

The good news is that none of the above is true. Surrender does not mean going backward, nor is it a suicidal act. It is actually a giant step forward on the spiritual journey and an opportunity to be more free and alive than we have ever imagined.

When Jesus said we must lose our lives in order to save them, he was speaking about the paradox of surrender. I am sure that most of his original listeners, including his disciples, did not understand what he meant. Surrender, like forgiveness, requires spiritual maturity in order to be truly appreciated and practiced, because it is paradoxical.

Paradox is an unavoidable reality on the journey to God. It is initially difficult because it appears contradictory and nonsensical. How can I lose my life in order to save my life? How can I achieve freedom by surrendering that freedom to a higher power? How can I control my weight by giving that control to something other than myself? These questions are all normal and rational and deserve answers. But they cannot be properly answered with normal logic. Spiritual logic is required.

Spiritual logic teaches us that the way of the ego (control) will never produce the results we want. In fact, it makes it very clear that control is pretty much an illusion. I lived under the thrall of this illusion the first half of my life. I was convinced I could control all manner of things . . . events, relationships, students, clients, children, my wife (on brief occasions) and my future.

I sought out the gurus of control and practiced every technique they espoused. I even convinced myself that I was producing meaningful results, because every once in a while things turned out the way I wanted. I naively thought I was the determining factor.

I thought I was in control of my life and my destiny—and I was wrong. I have since learned that my ability to make things happen is a grand illusion. And, to tell the truth, I am relieved. I was exhausting myself attempting to do the impossible, and I am tremendously thankful that I discovered this liberating truth: *I am not in control, and I don't need to be in control. God is in control, and that makes the whole thing O.K.*

Jesus taught me that surrendering my life to God will give me my life back. I heard that from the moment I was old enough to go to Bible school. It was far too sophisticated for a child's ears but I have finally reached an age that it makes sense.

*Control is an illusion. Surrender is the only sane alternative.* These sentences are my new mantras. I am more aware of their accuracy every day. I can't control my family, my clients, my workshop participants or my editors. I can't control the plumber, the gardener, the electrician, the auto repairman and the computer service guys.

I can't control the bugs that eat my favorite plants, the sunshine that nourishes them one day and burns them the next. I am totally beyond control of the ants and flies and roaches that periodically decide to call my home their home.

At the beginning of every week I look at my calendar and see what I have planned: the dates, times and goals. Then I laugh. I repeat my mantra because I know what is real. *Control is an illusion,* and surrender is the only sane alternative.

I am sure that anyone who has significant weight issues understands what I am saying. Very little in life is a better teacher about the illusion of control than the vicious cycle of weight gain and loss. We desperately want and need to lose weight, and every once in a while we do. We think maybe we can do it this time. We believe we are finally in control.

Then, bang, we wake up, stand on the scale and see the painful reality. The numbers are going up instead of down, and there is nothing we can do. Our weight has become a teacher that is pointing us to a bigger spiritual reality: *It is time to learn about surrender.*

If you are even a little like me, it takes a lot to get your attention and more to hold it. Maybe your weight is the thing that is required. Maybe your weight and your inability to control it will open a different kind of reality, the reality of surrender. If that happens, then you may come to see excess weight as one of the best friends you've had.

If you are ready to explore the release and peace that comes with surrender, you might start by praying this simple prayer. Pray it until something in your heart lets go. You don't need to know what it is, but you will feel it. When it happens, you will be on your way.

*"I realize that I cannot control my weight and my life. I let go and surrender to your love and care. Thy will be done."*

Then relax and let God do the rest. You were never in control anyway.

### Excess Weight: A Path to Self-Love

Most of us think of fat as the path to self-hate, and for many of us it is. We hate fat, and we hate ourselves for being fat. But there is another way to think about your weight problem that can change your perspective so dramatically, you will lose weight and learn to love yourself at the same time.

I realize that these words sound totally contrary to your daily experience. I am aware that excess weight may be a source of extreme pain and my suggestion may sound so absurd that it makes you angry. However, I would like to offer an alternative to that pain and a key to weight loss that may actually make sense.

In addition to having a God instinct and a natural predilection for prayer, human beings are designed to function best when they love themselves. Self-hate causes the human organism to self-destruct. Self-love causes the human organism to grow and prosper. You know it from personal experience. Self-love is good, and self-hate is not so good.

If fat causes us to hate ourselves, then losing weight should cause us to love ourselves. This assumption seems reasonable, but there is an unseen flaw here. The logic is backward. *Fat does not cause self-hate. Self-hate causes fat.*

I understand that being fat often contributes to a negative self-image, but it is not the ultimate cause. Fat is often the symptom. I use the word "often" because excess weight is not always a result of self-hate. There are exceptions, but in my experience they are few. In many cases, being significantly overweight is a symptom of low self-esteem and/or self-hate.

If self-hate is harmful to the healthy function of human beings and excess weight is a symptom of this painful and destructive disease, then fat can be a useful agent in our healing process. How could this be?

When I lived in Hawaii, I attended a heart-wrenching one-person play about the life of a priest named Damien who had given his life in service to the leper colony on the island of Molokai. During the course of his ministry, he contracted the terminal disease and finally died amid the very people he came to serve.

Damien left an account of his ministry and included a description of the progression of leprosy throughout his own body. The play included a portion of his journal in which he related his first awareness of the disease. He explained that he had a custom of soaking his feet in a pail of hot water at the end of a hard day. On this particular day, he poured the steaming water into a container and inserted his right foot. When he removed his foot a few minutes later, he realized that it was red and blistered.

He knew then that he had contracted the dread disease because he had lost feeling in his limb and was completely unaware of the extreme heat that had scorched his skin.

Father Damien's description about the quiet, but deadly, progress of leprosy has remained with me until this day. He made me aware of the supreme importance of pain and its essential role in the healing process. Without pain, we would be unaware of the existence of most dangerous diseases. Pain wakes us up and tells us to take notice. It bangs inconveniently and unceremoniously on the closed door of our unconsciousness and doesn't let up until it has our full attention. Pain often saves our lives. We would not be able to pass safely through a single day without its protection.

Hopefully, you are beginning to see my point about weight gain. Adding and sustaining significant weight can be both physically and emotionally painful. The pain is there for a reason. It is telling us to wake up to a deeper, more dangerous, condition that requires our immediate attention . . . self-hate.

Self-hate is one of the most far-reaching and destructive diseases we can contract. It can destroy our bodies, relationships, livelihoods and relationship with God. Left to its own devices, it eats away at every positive and life-giving aspect of our inner and outer being. We cannot afford to ignore its ultimately terminal effects, and we must learn to apply the only permanent cure . . . self-love.

Self-love, not weight loss, is the only cure for self-hate. Weight gain is often a clear symptom of self-hate, and as such it is our friend. It is pointing its unrelenting finger at the culprit. If we pay attention and act wisely, we can learn to apply the healing potion of self-love. Then we will not need the symptom of excess weight. In many cases, it begins to leave our bodies in a form of spontaneous remission. We lose weight without trying.

### Prayer and Self-Love

Every prayer is an act of self-love. Whether we are aware of it or not, every prayer we pray is a form of self-nurturing. Praying is a way of accessing and connecting to the most loving force in the universe. It is as beneficial to the human organism as breathing.

Prayer is a request for attention, care and love. This request comes directly from a part of us that cares about our essential well being . . . our self-love. Therefore, every prayer reinforces that deep-seated energy.

Self-hate cannot, by definition, create behavior that nurtures us. If prayer is nurturing, then it must originate in self-love. It cannot be otherwise. Since prayer is always an agent of self-love, then it makes sense to pray at all times. The more we pray, the more we fuel our capacity to love and value who we are. The more we increase our self-love and self-esteem, the easier it will become to sustain healthy attitudes and behaviors, including healthy eating patterns.

## *Excess Weight: A Guide To Healing Old Wounds*

Just as excess weight can lead us to a productive encounter with self-hate, it can also direct us to inner wounds that plague our everyday existence. Many obese persons, after listening to the deeper messages of their weight, can mark the beginning of weight gain with the onset of mental or emotional trauma. Childhood violence, sexual abuse, loss of a parent and emotional deprivation are only a few of the devastating experiences that can cause us to seek protection in food and layers of body fat.

It is important to know that significant symptoms have significant causes. People gain weight for a reason. People gain lots of weight for weighty reasons. Obesity is not the result of immaturity or simple lack of willpower. Its causes are as large as the excess pounds indicate. This fact is ultimately a blessing because it can direct us to the real sources of weight gain and will prevent us from settling for simplistic solutions. It should also create an atmosphere of compassion for one who suffers from chronic obesity.

If you are a person who is chronically overweight, you would do well to assume that it is a result of unhealed mental or emotional wounds. If you are willing to find the courage to explore and heal those wounds, you will almost certainly experience a change in your eating patterns. This process is not easy and is periodically painful, but the rewards can be enormous. I will offer one example.

Jackie, forty-two, came for a consultation and re-ported two major complaints. She was at least a hundred pounds overweight, and she had been plagued with the same nightmare two or three times a week since she was a child. She had the usual string of failures with diets and exercise and was almost in despair about losing weight. She had never been to a counselor for either problem and called me as a last resort.

After hearing her concerns, I asked Jackie to do two things. I requested that she pray daily for the strength to face the painful life experiences that were the source of her symptoms. I also asked her to begin a search for those wounds and to describe them to me in detail. I told her I would join her in praying for healing and guidance and that I was willing to hear every painful aspect of whatever her wound contained.

After a brief period of trust building, Jackie began to tell me a story that she had told only to her husband. She began by saying that she did not see what this had to do with weight gain, but she would share it anyway. She told me her nightmare.

It was a graphic account of her experience of her mother's suicide. Jackie was six years old and playing in her backyard when she heard a loud noise that seemed to come from her mother's bedroom. She ran in the back door and down a hall to her mother's room. Her mother looked as if she were asleep on the bed, so Jackie climbed up and tried to wake her.

When she touched her head, her hands became cov-ered with blood. Then she noticed the pistol in her mother's hand. Jackie got down from the bed and, covered in her mother's blood, ran screaming to her next-door neighbor. Here the dream ended.

Jackie was obviously traumatized by the event that stayed in her consciousness for over thirty-five years. But she had no idea it was related to her weight problem. She was actually surprised when I made the connection.

We talked about the dream for weeks. We prayed separately and together. First, she had a week with no nightmare, then two weeks, then the dream stopped altogether. Then she began to discover that her food binges were less frequent. She slowly lost weight. We continued to explore how her eating had become a way to manage the pain created by the violent loss of her mother.

She cried a lot. She raged at her mother. She found the courage to tell friends and trusted family members about her experience and her reaction to it. She prayed some more. She got thinner, happier and less depressed and she at last began to feel that she could manage her eating and her feelings.

Jackie's story is not unique. Many of us have horrible wounds that have never healed. We are the walking wounded. We often use food to assuage the pain because we are aware of no other choices. Sometimes, like Jackie, we finally look for help because the weight will not go away and we don't know what else to do.

Thank God for the weight that moves us to finally take care of our wounds. If it were not so obvious and so persistent, we might ignore our needs and live our lives without healing. If you are even vaguely like Jackie, I suggest that you pray this simple prayer and then follow the guidance it brings.

*"I am overweight and possibly wounded. Please guide me to compassionate and wise sources of healing."*

Pray with an open heart and mind, and the answer will come. You need and deserve healing. It will change your life.

### Excess Weight: A Lesson In Receiving

For centuries, Western society has suffered from a misinterpretation of the belief that it is better to give than to receive. We have made giving all-important and receiving insignificant or even bad. Many of us actually feel guilty when we have the opportunity to receive attention, care or love. We think we are being selfish and that being selfish means we don't care about others. We then try to live as if giving could exist without receiving. This is impossible and often results in destructive eating patterns.

Over the years, I have led numerous stress management workshops for nurses. These professional caregivers, so vital to our medical system, are consistently victimized by this erroneous attitude about giving. As a result, many suffer from symptoms of extreme stress, including weight problems.

Nurses often tell me they feel trapped in a difficult cycle. They give to their patients all day. Then they go home and give to their families. They find it almost impossible to take care of themselves or, God forbid, ask for help. If help is offered, they will automatically say, "No, thank you," and continue on without support. Food is often the only nurturing they allow themselves. It becomes the only giver they know, and eating is the only receiving they can accept.

Nurses are not alone in their inability to receive. Almost every overweight person has the same issue. Giving is easy, and receiving is almost out of the question. The problem is that giving and receiving are as related as breathing in and breathing out. One supports the other. What would happen if you tried to live only by breathing out?

Givers need to learn how to receive in order to continue giving without burning out or overeating. Weight gain is often a sign of an imbalance in our giving-receiving cycle. It can remind us that we have gone too far in one direction. For the overweight person, that almost always means too much giving and not enough receiving.

Excess weight can be a powerful message to those who are stuck in giving without receiving. It means that food is the only thing we allow ourselves to receive. We starve ourselves by refusing to ask for help or by rejecting the support that is offered. Then we eat to fill the emptiness that this behavior causes. If it were not for our weight, we might never pay attention and decide to seek help in another direction.

If you are not sure about your receiving abilities, you will benefit from the checklist I have included below.

### Are You a Good Receiver?

*"There are so many gifts*
*Still unopened from your birthday,*
*There are so many hand-crafted presents*
*That have been sent to you by God."*

—Hafiz

1. Do you find it easier to give than receive?
2. Do you get embarrassed when someone pays you a compliment?
3. Do you often confuse receiving with selfishness?
4. Has your religious training emphasized giving and neglected the idea of receiving?
5. Do you think God expects you to give without receiving?
6. Have you trained your coworkers and family members to see you as a perpetual giver?
7. Do you become verbally paralyzed when it is time to ask for help?
8. Is eating your major way of receiving?
9. Do you believe God wants to give to you because he loves you?
10. What would happen if you decided to ask for help in your life?

11. How could you practice being a better receiver today?
12. Are you willing to open your heart and mind to receive the love and care God wants to bring you?

Being chronically overweight is almost always a sign of an inability to receive. It is your body's reminder to pay attention to your needs and to allow others, God included, to help. All of us could use improvement in this area. We would all benefit from the following prayer.

> *"Gracious and giving God, open my heart and mind so I can receive and enjoy today all the love and support that you want to offer me."*

---

*What if God made giving and receiving identical to breathing? What if one supports and replenishes the other? What if receiving was as easy as breathing in? Would you pray for the ability to breathe more deeply?*

---

### Excess Weight: A Path to Loving Your Body

Believe it or not, being overweight is an opportunity to learn to love your body. Judeo-Christian tradition teaches that God made the human body and called it good. Christians also believe that the body is the temple of the Holy Spirit. Therefore, both traditions are emphatic about the value and significance of the physical body. God gave us our bodies, and God intends us to love and enjoy those bodies. Body love is not contrary to the two major religious influences of Western society.

But body love is not prevalent in America. We are obsessed with our bodies, but obsession is not love. In fact, it is exactly the opposite. We are obsessed with our bodies because we *hate* them. Body hate is more the rule than body love. We are constantly trying to change the way we look from the tops of our balding heads to our eyes, noses, throats, stomachs, buttocks and feet. We hate the slightest indication of fat or age, so we literally attack our bodies if any sign of either shows up.

Even though our religious traditions set a good precedent for body love, we seem to have gone in the opposite direction. We don't accept or appreciate our bodies; we hate them and are ingenious in our techniques for changing them. It is no wonder that the majority of us are fat. Our bodies are in rebellion. They hate being hated, and they resist every effort we make to reject or change them.

If you want to lose weight, you will have to learn to love your body. Hate is never an effective motivator for change. Hate increases resistance. It generates mistrust and misunderstanding. Body hate will almost certainly guarantee that you will stay fat. If you want to lose weight, you will have to learn to love your body.

To learn body love, we must see our weight through inner, spiritual eyes. The eyes of the world have taught us to judge and condemn our bodies. Our inner eyes will help us achieve a different and more compassionate perspective. We need to see our weight not as a bad thing, but as our body's consistent cry for help; the greater the weight, the more intense the cry.

Imagine that I am right about this. Your excess weight is your body's way of saying, "Help. I am in trouble, and I need you to listen." It cries out to you every moment of every day. This means that your weight is not your enemy. It is not a torture technique that an unfriendly body has invented. Your excess weight is like a white flag on the field of battle. It is a request for an end to the conflict.

Our society has taught us to be insensitive to the cries of our bodies. Too often, we see the white flag of surrender and open fire. This leaves our wounded and misunderstood bodies with no alternative but to increase their attempts to get our compassionate attention. They usually accomplish that through diabetes, high blood pressure, strokes, heart attacks and other weight-related white flags.

If we change our perspective and view our excess weight as our body's way of asking for our help, we will almost immediately experience an increasing compassion for its suffering. That compassion is the beginning of body love, and it will provide us with the only real and lasting motivation for body care and weight loss. If you want to learn to love your body, you might begin by praying this prayer.

*"I know, dear Creator, that you made my body. Open my heart to my body's cries and teach me to love it even as you do."*

> *What if your body was created to be your friend? What if excess weight is your friend's cry for help? What would you pray for then?*

## Excess Weight: A Constant Guide to Growth

My experience with my own and my clients' weight issues has convinced me that weight can be a wonderful agent for both personal and spiritual growth. The decision is ours. We can remain unhappy and powerless victims of our society's obsessive fat-hate or we can pray for a new and transforming vision of our bodies and their invitations to growth.

We need all the help we can get on our lifelong journey to God. It is time to accept the intimate and attentive care that our bodies are offering us. Once we see our weight through compassionate eyes, we will begin to see the many lessons that it wants to teach us. Weight loss will be only one of the gifts we will receive.

> *"Thank you, dear wise and compassionate Creator, for giving me a body that always supports my growth and healing. Thank you for every lesson and gift that it brings me."*

*Three*

# A NEW VISION OF WEIGHT LOSS AND THE LIBERATION OF PRAYER

———— ⌾⌾ ————

*"There is a hidden love-center*
*in human beings that you will discover and savor*
*and nourish yourself with. That will be your food . . .*

*Stop swimming so hard,*
*and climb in the boat*
*with Noah."*

—Jelaludin Rumi

———— ⌾⌾ ————

*Loaves and Fishes*

*"This is not*
*the age of information.*

*This is not*
*the age of information.*

*Forget the news,*
*and the radio,*
*and the blurred screen.*

*This is the time*
*of loaves*
*and fishes.*

*People are hungry,*
*and one good word is bread*
*for a thousand."*

—David Whyte

Obesity is an American plague. Over 55 percent of us are overweight and the number is growing, along with our waistlines, cholesterol levels and bypass surgeries. Our weight dulls us, drugs us, makes many of us ill and often kills us. We are being buried under a mountain of fat, and we are screaming for help. We spend enormous amounts of money every year on thousands of programs that promise quick, easy and lasting weight loss. And still we get fatter.

I have not overstated my case when I use the phrase "the American plague." We suffer emotionally, physically, mentally and spiritually from obesity. Being overweight is not simply a matter of vanity. For many of us, it significantly restricts the quality, expression and length of our lives. We are overweight and in pain. We are desperate, often hopeless and confused. We are crying out for a light to lead us out of the dark forest of food abuse and addiction. Sadly, we are only being led by the blind.

I am convinced, therefore, that we need a new vision of the entire weight-loss process; a vision that has both breadth and depth and takes all the relevant issues into consideration. To my knowledge, there is not a program or process that does this. Most weight-loss programs focus on surface issues—diet and exercise— and ignore the deeper and more crucial factors that actually control eating patterns. Almost every program avoids or trivializes the central issue of spirituality, and the few that do not are so sectarian they offend more than they include.

I am also convinced that this plague that so painfully besets us can become an agent of liberation. We can view and experience it through the pharaoh's horrified eyes or the hopeful hearts of the enslaved Hebrew tribes. It can kill us as the angel of death killed the firstborn of the Egyptians or it can lead us to a new and transformed existence. It is our choice.

We will get to the promised land of weight loss only if we develop a new and well-balanced vision that includes all the essential ingredients. We cannot afford to ignore, avoid or trivialize any of them. Each must have its recognition and consideration, and each must be allowed to relate to the others.

I have briefly outlined the four factors I consider to be essential to a well-balanced weight-loss process. I pray that everyone in the weight-loss community will use these four categories to evaluate and upgrade their programs. There are experts in each of the four who can make wonderful contributions to the other three. It is time we joined hands and created meaningful solutions that can benefit us all.

The problem with proposed solutions for problems is that we look at what is obvious and assume we have the answer. The traditional reaction to being overweight is to assume too much food and too little exercise caused the weight gain; therefore we need to simply reverse that process and we will become thin.

After a thousand failures, we still act as if this assumption is valid. This behavior can only be called neurotic—

we constantly repeat an action and expect a different result each time. If I hit myself over the head with a hammer, I will split my skull. It doesn't matter if I change the color of the grip or the position of my fingers. After fifty years of headaches, it is time to put down the hammer and look for better alternatives to weight loss.

> *What if your body was your greatest spiritual asset? How would you treat it, and what prayer would you pray for it?*

### Meaningful Weight Loss—Four Essential Factors

I believe there are four basic ingredients in every effective weight-loss process. To achieve meaningful and lasting weight loss, all four must be satisfied. Contrary to popular opinion, we need to attend to the least obvious first. Dieting and exercise may need to wait until we confront and explore the two deeper, more complex, factors.

Each of the factors is interdependent. If one is neglected, it affects and creates symptoms in each of the other areas. Weight loss cannot be sustained unless all four factors are balanced.

Anyone can lose weight through initial attention to any one of the four essential areas. Most weight-loss programs are built on this reality. But almost no one can sustain weight loss this way. Sooner or later, the other three factors assert their needs and the weight returns. Only an integrated approach will produce lasting results. We must include all four factors.

### Factor One—Spirituality.

> *"All talents of God are within you.*
>
> *How could this be otherwise*
> *When your soul*
> *Derived from His*
> *Genes!"*

—Hafiz

I believe that humans are naturally spiritual. We have a God instinct. This instinct is not peripheral to our health and well-being—it is essential. If we ignore or trivialize it, we decompensate and suffer. One of the most common symptoms of spiritual neglect is obesity.

We may exercise and diet religiously, but sooner or later our spiritual needs will assert themselves and we will be unable to maintain our weight managing disciplines. We may also delve deeply into our emotional past and confront our worst psychological traumas, but without spiritual support and inspiration we may find ourselves lost in a forest of cynicism and meaninglessness. Weight gain is sure to follow.

Each of us has spiritual needs. We must learn to attend to them and integrate them into our daily existence.

Simply becoming religious is not the answer. We must find authentic spiritual nurturing that speaks directly to our particular consciousness and life situation. There are no absolute formulas for this.

I am sure there are many who wish I would offer one path as the solution for all. I wish it were that easy, but it is my experience that each of us has major differences. I would rather leave this to you and your prayers for God's guidance in your life. I am simply the voice that reminds you to pray, not the one who answers them.

Every balanced weight-loss program will have a clear and developed spiritual component. That component will support and facilitate the well-being of the other three and will receive the same.

### Factors Two and Three—Mental and Emotional Issues

I have placed these two factors together because they are extremely difficult to separate. Whether we separate them or not, they are essential to the weight-loss process. Willpower and self-discipline will almost always run screaming out the door when confronted with the monsters of deep psychological complexes.

Everyone has unresolved inner issues, and everyone is affected in significant ways by these powerful forces of the psyche. No one is exempt. Anyone who attempts to lose weight will eventually meet these forces, and those who are unprepared will be overwhelmed by their power.

An integrated and balanced weight-loss process will provide structures and techniques that guide its participants into and through their mental and emotional jungles. Self-hate, body hate, abuse of all kinds, depression, anxiety, rage, loneliness and loss are only a few of the issues and energies that control our eating patterns. If they are not addressed and healed or managed, we cannot expect to sustain healthy and nurturing behaviors. Programs that promise weight loss without attending to these factors are irresponsible and naive and ultimately add to the despair and low self-esteem of chronically obese persons.

### Factor Four—The Physical Body

Everyone knows that diet and exercise are essential to weight loss. There are many superb exercise and diet programs that have been developed by creative and experienced professionals. We do not lack information or expertise in these areas, and we should draw on the skills and wisdom of these individuals. They have not been ineffective because they are incompetent but because of what they did not include.

The majority of the weight-loss community is composed of diet and exercise programs, and it is time they faced the sad, but obvious, reality: They have not solved the problem. Ultimately, they all fail and that failure cannot be blamed on lack of self-discipline or commitment of their participants.

Something vital is missing from their programs, and that something makes all the difference. Three vital factors (spiritual, mental and emotional) must be conjoined with the valuable and necessary physical factor before success can be achieved.

Weight-loss programs need a new vision to become viable options to anyone who is overweight. That vision must be bigger and deeper than anything currently available. It must include and integrate the four basic factors or systems that comprise human existence. We must recognize and nurture our spiritual, mental, emotional and physical selves so we can live and eat with health and enthusiasm.

A new and comprehensive vision of weight loss will change our perspective. We will lose our view of weight gain as a plague and begin to see it as a path to a transformed sense of our bodies, our inner selves, of prayer and of God. It is up to us to make the choice. I invite you to pray with me for that end.

> *What if weight gain was God's way of getting your attention and an invitation to growth and love? How would you feel about being fat, and how then would you pray?*

## The Liberation of Prayer

> *"It's not me that's glorified in acts of worship.*
> *It's the worshipers! I don't hear the words*
> *that they say. I look inside at the humility.*

## The Prayer Diet

*That broken-open lowliness is the reality,*
*not the language! Forget phraseology.*
*I want burning, burning . . .*

*Inside the Kaaba,*
*it doesn't matter which direction you point*
*your prayer rug!*

*The ocean diver doesn't need snowshoes!*
*The love-religion has no code or doctrine.*
*Only God."*

—Jelaludin Rumi

*For millennia, prayer has been held hostage by organized re-*
*ligion.* From the days of the pharaohs, the religion of the
day has dictated the prayers of the day. Too often, prayer
has been taught as a formula that must be mixed properly
in order to produce desired results. In many cases, the
improper use of prayer words or phrases has been considered blasphemy and could lead to imprisonment or
death.

Excessive attention to prayer rules, rituals and dogma
has taken prayer out of the hands of those who pray into
the hands of religious professionals. It is no wonder so
many people do not pray or are not at ease with the
prayers they use.

Recently, I watched a popular television drama in
which a central figure lay in a coma in an intensive care

unit. Friends and family surrounded her bed, and one individual suggested they pray together. Everyone joined hands, bowed their heads, closed their eyes and said nothing. The scene ended, and the episode was over.

I am fully aware that the actors were not given prayer lines because there is great fear of being religiously incorrect. A silent prayer is the safest prayer. But prayer is not about safety; it is about passion, heart, care and love. Yet no one spoke for the healing of their dying friend. Something is wrong with this picture.

It is sad testimony to the strange impotence of the religious community that television can portray hundreds of acts of sex and violence every hour of every day, but no one is allowed to pray out loud in prime time. I am not blaming the entertainment community for this craziness. They are not responsible for our society's insanity about prayer and religious differences. We, the viewers, would much rather see a man have part of his brain eaten or a woman raped than hear a prayer prayed "incorrectly."

This dogmatically restrictive attitude is as old as prayer itself and is the reason Rumi spoke to it so eloquently 750 years ago. He knew what every mystic of every religious tradition knows: that authentic prayer has no sacred formula except the "burning" in the heart of the one who prays. Words have little importance and certainly do not control or manipulate God's ability to respond.

I do not consider prayer to be a human right. I see it as part of human instinct. It is more basic than a right, which can be taken away. It is an attribute of the God instinct that is present in every one of us. Prayer is like breathing: natural and normal. Do religious pundits have the power or the right to tell us when and how we can inhale and exhale? Do we sin if we breathe deeply or quickly? What if we hold our breath? Could there be a breathing ritual that separates the righteous from the unrighteous? I hope not.

Let's return to the TV drama and consider a revised scenario. What if each person had been allowed to pray an individual heartfelt prayer for the friend? What if each person's love and fear and hope and care had been prayed out loud?

What if each one had used unique words and phrases to talk intimately with God? I'll tell you what would have happened. From California to the Carolinas, there would not have been a dry eye or a closed heart. Every viewer would have been touched and inspired. America would have prayed out loud together and it would have been O.K.

It is time for us to liberate prayer from its rigid religious inhibitions. We can learn to pray as normally and naturally as we breathe. We can pray anywhere and everywhere, about everything and anything. We can use the words and phrases that emerge from our burning hearts and souls without fear that God will object or recoil.

For many of us, our frustration and pain about weight gain is a powerful motivation to pray. It brings us to the "broken-open lowliness" that Rumi describes above. We know that we have met a power greater than ourselves and must call out humbly to an even larger power for healing. At this point, prayer is natural and should not require religiously correct phraseology. An infant crying in the night does not need words to be heard clearly by an ever-attentive mother.

I have always felt that God's greatest miracle is his ability to use ordinary events in extraordinary ways. What could be more ordinary than fat? What could be more a part of our everyday existence than weight loss and gain? The majority of us think about it every single day. What could be a better vehicle for God's mercy and guidance than something that touches so many of us so often? What could be a more persistent call to prayer than our frustration and desperation about our weight?

I believe that prayer needs to be a natural and normal part of our lives. I know it can change our body weight and the more painful weight in our hearts. It can lift us, inspire us, heal us and draw us ever closer to the true source of all being. To do this, prayer must be liberated from restriction and dogma and be returned to its rightful place at the center of every human heart. Prayer is the most human act we can perform.

> *May God bless you, and may Grace draw you ever closer with each prayer that you pray.*

*"This is the time*
*For you to compute the impossibility*
*That there is anything but Grace.*

*Now is the season to know*
*That everything is Sacred."*

—Hafiz

## Four

# THE DIETER'S PRAYER

---

*"I was a tiny bug. Now a mountain.*
*I was left behind. Now honored at the head.*

*You healed my wounded hunger and anger,*
*and made me a poet who sings about joy."*

—Jelaludin Rumi

---

I did not know that I was a writer until I met my second (and current) wife. We met, and something exploded inside. I am, to this day, inadequate to the task of describing it accurately. I can say that our initial romance was spiritual because it remains ineffable, but it was also emotional, mental and deeply physical. I have often referred to our connection as a meeting of soul mates. Whatever the definition, I was changed dramatically by the encounter and ensuing relationship.

From the moment we met, I felt a rising tide of awareness that something was about to be liberated within me. Her presence, her energy, her directness, her passion, her enthusiasm and her love seemed to pop open the door of a cage I had kept my best self in for years. Part of what emerged was my ability to write.

It was not surprising that my first venture into heart-directed writing was love letters and poems to her. Thankfully, I wrote them in a hardbound journal and they have survived the last twenty-seven years intact. Objectively, they are the work of a beginner, but emotionally they are clear testimony to a love that has liberated and sustained me to this day.

As I wrote to her, I began to experience writing as a powerfully creative act. I had never thought of myself as creative, but after writing two or three love letters I knew I had begun a process that would become a natural and necessary part of my life.

We met in 1973, and for the next ten years I wrote sporadically in my journal and infrequent articles for local magazines and papers. In 1984, I self-published a small book of psychological and spiritual insights. I was too intimidated and insecure to risk the almost certain rejection of real publishing companies, so I printed them myself.

I struggled with my partially liberated drive to write for six more years until we moved to Florida, and then I began to write in earnest. Over the next eight years, I wrote three books. I was blessed to find two separate literary agents who energetically proposed two of my productions to all the major publishers. Everyone said no.

I was confused and frustrated by these negative developments. I thought my work was well-written and timely. I knew I was a writer, and I believed God was directing me to write. He had given me this gift, and I was certain he wanted me to use it. He had even introduced me to two successful and respected agents who were enthusiastic about my work. But they were unable to open one door to a publisher.

I had many long and emotional talks with my wife about what was happening. With her wise encouragement, I began to let go and allow myself to trust that things would happen as they needed to and not at my direction. I focused my energy on my counseling practice and reminded myself that letting go was the order of the day.

I suppose I should have understood the frustrating process of waiting, hoping and not knowing. It is essential and common for a spiritual journey. I was not lost or forgotten by God. I had not drifted off the path. I was simply being prepared in ways that I could not see. But I was not patient, and I often complained to God about it.

*"Listen, is there something you can do to help me out here? I have written three books, and they are all good. You know that, and I know that. I have even found two agents. You of all beings know how hard that is. Why did you give me agents if they were going to be ineffective and unsuccessful? Am I missing something here? If I am, please tell me because I want to get on with this thing."*

Sometimes complaining to God can be cathartic. God can take it, and he never seems to lose his patience. For me, it is an honest expression of real feelings. I am not proud of these sessions, but who would I be kidding if I did not admit to them? Sometimes I am this way and thank God for his understanding. I usually get better after a session and then am able to pray a deeper and more meaningful prayer.

*"O.K. I am calmer now. I guess that the best thing to do now is trust and let go. I always have great resistance to this part, but I really love it when I am finally able. I surrender to your wisdom and your care. I surrender to your vision and your time. I let go into your love. I surrender, and I am at peace in that surrender."*

On occasion, I pray the prayer that is actually the only prayer that a true friend of God needs: *Thy will be done.* But usually I am less trusting and therefore more verbose. Either way, I assume that God hears the real heart message that is often buried under my words.

I have realized over the years that I seldom use a name for God when I begin a prayer. This is not a sign of disrespect but an indication of intimacy. When I telephone my wife every day from my office, I do not use her first name when I say hello. We speak so often that I am sure she recognizes my voice as I do hers. My conversations with God are even more frequent, and the connection is seldom broken for long. Saying "Lord" or "Dear God" or "Father in heaven" is perfectly appropriate, but it most often feels stilted and strained to me. So I just talk, either silently or out loud, and between prayers I try to listen to him as carefully as he does to me.

### The Prediction

Near the end of 1999, my wife and I went to Orlando, Florida, for a long weekend, and I had a surprising encounter with a psychic.

Psychics live and work on the edge of acceptability in American society. They are condemned as agents of evil by some conservative religious groups. In other circles, presidential and otherwise, they are consulted before any major life decision is made.

I prefer to categorize psychics with attorneys, physicians, psychotherapists and clergy. Some are competent, many are average and nondescript, a few are charlatans and con artists and some (a real but definite minority) have a mysteriously accurate connection to a nonordinary reality. Contact with those in the last group can be helpful, healing and enlightening. I have been blessed to encounter at least three of these.

This particular trip to Orlando was for rest and relaxation, but we especially wanted to visit a small village about thirty miles north of the city called Casadaga. I had been told a wonderful story about this "psychic center" by a client some years before and had immediately placed it on our "Things To Do When in Orlando" list. This weekend, we actually found our way there. A former client named Bob had brought me to this amazing place.

## Bob's Story

About four years earlier I had a thirty-five-year-old client named Bob (not his real name) who had had an unusually abusive father. His father had died when Bob was eighteen, leaving him alone to heal his painful and life-shaping wounds. Since his father's death, the young man had traveled from one therapist to another attempting to shed the burden of his dysfunctional parent's legacy. He had made little progress and remained very much the victim of his ongoing rage and hurt.

One afternoon, Bob walked into my office with the brightest and most uncharacteristic smile I had ever seen. He said he had a miracle story to tell me.

Bob said his wife had heard of a village north of Orlando (Casadaga) that had been a center for spiritualism and psychics for over fifty years. They decided to visit it, and upon arriving, walked into a small book-and-gift store near the town's only stoplight. On a wall they saw a list of local psychics. Bob had no idea who to select, so he said a quiet prayer for guidance and picked one with an appealing name. He made a phone call and was given an immediate appointment.

Bob went to the psychic's office and sat down in front of a normal-looking, middle-aged woman who said, *"Don't tell me anything about yourself. Just let me hold your hand for a moment."* Bob complied. The woman touched his hand, closed her eyes and said a prayer asking for God to bless him and their meeting and to guide her as she worked. Then she sat back in her chair and began to talk.

She told Bob that someone who "had made his transition" (psychic language for having died) was with her and had a message for Bob. She described the person physically and spoke his first name. Bob was astounded because she used his father's name, which was very uncommon, and described him exactly as Bob had known him.

Then she delivered the message, and Bob began to cry. She said this man wanted Bob to know he had been extremely hurtful to Bob when Bob was a child. He said he was ashamed and sorry for what he had done and that he loved his son deeply and needed his forgiveness.

Bob cried again as he related this amazing and moving story. He said nothing had done more to heal his heart and his relationship with his dead father than this encounter. He still did not understand what had happened, but was deeply grateful for the experience. I was impressed with Bob's story and decided to make my own trip to Casadaga.

## My Story

My wife and I arrived in Casadaga in much the same fashion as Bob. We approached the lists of psychics and selected a name. I did not remember the name of the person Bob had seen, so I prayed a simple prayer. *"Give us some guidance here. I have no idea how to do this or how to make a good selection. Please lead us to the right person today."* We called, made an appointment and drove around the block to the psychic's house.

When I sat with the woman we had chosen, she began with a prayer just like the one Bob had related. Then she touched my hand and began to talk. Over the course of an hour she told me many things that were interesting and helpful, but one thing in particular seemed absurd. I filed it in my memory and shared it with my wife on the ride home.

The psychic told me that I would be doing quite a bit of writing in the next year and for years to come. I was pleased to hear that but was not impressed. Other psychics had told me that I was a creative type and should be a writer. Then she made a comment that I thought was totally off base. She said that I would be writing for the Internet and that it would change my life in some significant ways.

The woman clearly had more faith in her vision of my future than I did. But then, she did not know that in 1999, I was a computer illiterate. My wife had just bought our first system a few months before, and we waited weeks to unpack it. I barely knew how to connect to the Internet, and I was a novice, ten-words-a-minute, typist.

I checked my e-mail once every seven or eight days and clearly preferred phone messages. I saw no use for the computer as a writing tool, and I had no intention of becoming an expert, much less a nerd. I thought the woman had momentarily confused me with someone else, and I was happy when she went on to more relevant and acceptable predictions. One year later, in the midst of my weekly work with eDiets.com, I decided she was a genius.

I have included these stories about psychics for a particular purpose. Psychic guidance and prediction is out of the mainstream of American thinking. According to the ever-present polls, less than 20 percent of us have ever been to a psychic. I am not suggesting that the number should rise or that psychic guidance is necessary for spiritual growth. I am saying that God often answers prayer in unpredictable and mysterious ways. He frequently speaks to us through people, situations and experiences that are outside our expectations. If we close our minds and rigidly limit the channels we listen to, we run the risk of missing his message altogether. This is particularly relevant to praying about weight loss.

## EDiets.com and the Internet

When my friend, John McGran, called and asked me to write an article for his new employer, I was excited but had no expectation of an ongoing relationship. Initially, I suggested five pieces about extreme stress because I did not see myself as a weight-loss writer. But the accuracy of my perception was not necessary; only my cooperation was needed. God was busy answering my prayer to use me fully and completely, and it did not matter that I was currently unaware of His intentions.

The first articles were so well received, John invited me to write a weekly column. My enthusiasm increased, and I suggested that we name the column "Coyote Wisdom" after one of my books that was still in "the rejection process." Within a month, I had settled into the flow of one article per week, and I began to receive dozens of e-mails from readers who found my comments and ideas useful.

I quickly began to experience one of the most special gifts of the Internet—a deep sense of connection to people all over the world. I had heard much to the contrary about the effects of this new electronic world. Many critics of the Internet complain about its purported damage to meaningful interpersonal relationships, but my experience has been just the opposite.

I felt an immediate and even intimate awareness of my readers and their concerns. It was and is as powerful for me as any one-on-one, in-the-flesh counseling session.

My commitment to my column increased dramatically as I became aware of the real-life individuals who were reading my work and following my suggestions. Feedback was immediate and very personal. I would write an article about powerful emotions that cause us to overeat, and I would begin receiving e-mails about its usefulness within minutes after it appeared on the eDiets Web site.

Readers openly shared their painful struggles with weight and body image, relationships and self-hate and failures and successes. I was touched and began to see this work as a direct answer to my prayer. I was being used, and it felt great.

I began to pray an old prayer with a new level of intensity and frequency.

*"I need guidance. I need to be led to ideas and attitudes and techniques that will help my readers. Speak to me and make me aware of what works here. Don't let me get out of touch with what is wanted and needed. Don't let me become pedantic, patronizing or impersonal. Teach me to communicate with compassion and understanding and help me to stay open to the real needs of my readers."*

I have prayed this prayer daily for over a year, and I am never disappointed. Ideas, information, guidelines, techniques and understanding flow into my awareness at an incredible rate. I am never at a loss and, to date, have not had a moment of writer's block. The Prayer Diet experiment was one of the many answers to my prayers.

One evening in early July of 2000, I was walking our

dogs. I enjoy the experience and have come to view it as a time to receive answers to my prayers for writing ideas. We walk together three to five times a week, and I have never returned from our half-hour stroll without at least one or more ideas for an article.

Our regular turnaround point is a churchyard. It was here on the turf that I have seldom walked over the last 30 years that the idea of a Prayer Diet came to me. I was surprised at the venue and the idea because I have not walked the normal or traditional path of one so deeply and clearly called to the ministry. My lifestyle (my wife is Jewish) and my work as a counselor, organizational consultant and seminar leader have taken me outside the boundaries of the organized church, and I have often remarked half-seriously that my calling was to the "unchurched."

Since 1972, when I finished a two-year stint as assistant pastor of a small Congregationalist church outside of Boston, I have not been a regular member of a single congregation. Over the years, I have preached in numerous services at various locations but never with relish and not once with a feeling of being at home. My congregation has been populated by unbelievers and agnostics, the disaffected and disillusioned, the independent and rebellious and especially those who have been wounded by the organized church.

It was there, amid their anger, loneliness and courageous searching, that I found myself closest to God. It is ironic, therefore, that God gave me such a wonderful idea with such a traditional subject as prayer on the grounds of a church. I have always known that God has a sense of humor. I am convinced that this was one of his playful moments.

## The Prayer Diet Article

> *What if you pray for weight loss and your prayer is answered to the exact pound you requested? What will you do then?*

In mid-July, my editor ran my article entitled "The Prayer Diet." I was anxious about the reception it would get. EDiets is not a religious diet center, and even though I am never censored in my subject matter, I had some concern about the membership's reaction. Within hours, I knew my anxiety was unfounded and that something extraordinary was happening.

I was still writing one column a week. I was accustomed to receiving twenty to thirty e-mails a day. The day eDiets published the Prayer Diet article, I received over 1,000 e-mails from readers eager to participate in the experiment I proposed. The next day, another thousand arrived and they continued to pour in until the article had to be taken off-line and placed into the archives. The total number of e-mails about the Prayer Diet was over 5,000. I was astounded.

More touching and impressive than the numbers were the messages contained in almost every e-mail. I have included excerpts below. These are representative of the many thousands I have received since. The first message has been stated in one form or another in over 30 percent of the e-mails I have received.

> *"I am a person who believes in the power of prayer, but I never thought of praying for weight loss. Thank you so much for reminding me that God cares about every part of my life."*

> *"Please include me in the prayer experiment. I am 150 pounds overweight, and nothing else has worked. Thank you for the hope."*

> *"What a wonderful idea! I want to thank you and eDiets for bringing spirituality to your diet program."*

> *"I have never heard of such a thing, but I am willing to try anything to lose this weight. Maybe it will work."*

> *"I want to try the prayer experiment, but I am not sure I have the faith. Can I try it anyway? Please help me."* (I wrote back immediately and said yes.)

> *"This is such a fantastic idea. I need to lose only 15 pounds. Is it O.K. to pray for that small amount?"* (Yes.)

> *"May God bless you for reminding us that he cares. I will start praying today."*

> *"I have never prayed about anything, but I want to start with this. I am so sick of being fat. God help me."*

*"I am a Christian, a Jew, a Muslim, a Buddhist, a Sufi, a Baha'i, a New Ager, an agnostic, an atheist. Can I pray for weight loss?"* (Yes!)

The initial Prayer Diet experiment was very simple. I asked participants to pray the Dieter's Prayer (described below) three times a day for two weeks and then e-mail me the results.

I did not try to set up a scientifically controlled experiment and I did not tell participants to stop any diet program they were on. I simply asked them to pray. Many of the e-mailers told me, however, that they were "diet free" except for the Prayer Diet. I joined the experiment myself and prayed the prayer every day.

Two weeks later, people began to respond. Once again, I was amazed. Here are some messages I received.

*"Thank God, I lost 7 pounds! I am so thrilled, and I feel so loved and cared about."*

*"I prayed the prayer every day for two weeks, and I lost 3 pounds. I will continue to pray. God has taken away more than just weight from my body. Thank you for the experiment."*

*"A miracle has occurred in my life. I lost 15 pounds by praying! Now I will be praying about everything. Thank you, thank you, thank you."*

*"I prayed every day for two weeks, and I did not lose any weight. But I have never felt more at peace. I will try to keep on praying, if only for the peace of mind it gives me."*

*"Guess what? This thing works. I lost 5 pounds, and have told every one of my friends to start praying. Is God great or what?"*

*"I have always prayed about almost everything. I believe in the power of prayer. Thank you for reminding me that I can pray about weight loss also. I lost 4 lbs."*

*"I am so thankful for the opportunity to pray this prayer. It has changed my life. Not only did it cause me to lose 4 pounds, but I feel God's presence more than I have ever felt it. I am not alone."*

*"When I started your experiment, I thought prayer was a waste of time. I only tried it because I was desperate. Nothing else has worked. Now, believe it or not, I am a believer. I lost 5 pounds!!! I am still praying."*

*"When I first read your article about prayer, I got angry. I have been mad at God for years for making me fat. I have been fat since I was a child, and I hate it. Why should I ask God to take away something that he gave me to start? But this time something made me pray. I lost 6 pounds in two weeks, and I am praying to God every day to help me lose the rest. Today I am not so angry at him."*

*"I have only prayed the Diet Prayer for three days so far, but I had to write and tell you that I have already lost 2.5 pounds! I don't know what will happen next, but I am already a believer. God bless."*

*"I have just finished one of the most amazing experiences of my life. I prayed about losing weight. I lost weight (5 pounds) and began to wake up to my eating habits in a way I have never been aware of. It was as if the prayer opened my eyes. I can see what I am doing to myself. Thank God, and thank you for the prayer."*

The number of e-mails that report weight loss results has continued to rise. I receive reports from individuals every week who have just discovered the article and want to join and from others who have just finished the two-week experiment. To date, I have received over 2,000 reports from people who faithfully completed the process.

## THE PRAYER DIET RESULTS TO DATE

Current number of Prayer Diet participants = 5,000+
Current number of Prayer Diet respondents = 2,000+
Average weight loss reported = 4.5 pounds over two weeks
Highest weight loss reported = 15 pounds over two weeks
Lowest weight loss reported = 0 pounds over two weeks

I am very excited about these results. The average loss of 4.5 pounds over two weeks is almost exactly what eDiets recommends for long-term weight loss. Anything higher than two or three pounds per week is not considered appropriate, desirable or healthy. These results have convinced me that long-term prayer will produce long-term weight loss, and I hope this book will encourage more individuals to participate in an ongoing prayer process.

Since I am not accustomed to conducting studies such as this, I do not know if 2,000 respondents out of 5,000 participants who began the experiment is a high or low number. I suspect that under the circumstances it is high. The entire process was created and supported by only one small article that was published on the eDiets Internet site for three days. Participants were given simple directions with no underlying context or guidance. I suppose the results achieved are more testimony to the amazing power of prayer.

I am hopeful that the information, guidelines, additional prayers and inspiration contained in this book will encourage many more readers to join the Prayer Diet process and sustain those prayers over a longer period of time. The results could be miraculous.

### The Prayer Diet—Joining the Experiment

To participate in the Prayer Diet, you need to do only the following:

1. *Pray the Dieter's Prayer three times a day.* I suggest you pray before breakfast, lunch and dinner. You may

pray the prayer more than three times if you like. As you pray the prayer, think about its deeper meaning. Remember that this prayer is not a magic formula. The words are not perfect or especially powerful in and of themselves. God is listening to the message in your heart. That is what really matters.

2. *Open yourself to receive whatever answers and guidance God wants to give you.* Weight loss is your first interest, but allow God to give you more than that. Prayer is a mystery and can bring much more than you may imagine.

3. *Write the Dieter's Prayer on a card and place it where you will encounter it throughout the day.* People report to me they carry the prayer in their pockets, appointment books, taped to their refrigerators, in their cars and on their computers. Place it where you feel comfortable. Simply seeing it will remind you of its purpose and return you to a prayerful frame of mind.

4. *If possible, find friends or family members to join the Prayer Diet with you.* This step is not a requirement, but everyone does better with support.

---

### THE DIETER'S PRAYER

*DEAR GOD (DIVINE PRESENCE):*
*I surrender my body and my weight loss to your divine care and love.*
*I ask that you remove all excess and unnecessary weight from my body.*
*Return my body to its most healthy and balanced state.*
*Give me eating habits that support my health and life energy.*
*And finally, teach me to love my body and to care for it from this day forth.*
*Amen.*

---

You may send me the results of your prayer experiment after thirty or sixty days. My contact addresses are listed at the end of the book. I am also praying for you.

### The Dieter's Prayer—How It Works

The Dieter's Prayer contains six elements that deserve clarification. Each one contributes to the growth and health of the one who prays.

1. *Surrender.* Surrender is essential to the process of prayer and spiritual growth. It provides release from the constrictions and severe limitations that our egos create. It frees us from the natural human desire to control everything in our lives. It places us in the best position to receive God's answers in the form he sees fit. And, finally, it gives us an in-

creasing sense of inner peace and trust in a presence and care greater than ourselves.

2. *Divine care and love.* It is important to remember who and what we are praying to. Our prayer does not emerge from our hearts and fly out into the nothingness of space. It is heard without hesitation by a God who cares unconditionally about every aspect of our lives and bodies. This God is as close to us as our own heartbeat. This God wants to become our most intimate companion, guide and healer. This God, once properly introduced, is a God we can love without fear or reservation.

3. *Unnecessary body weight.* The amount of weight lost must be up to God, not us. Far too many of us are dominated by unhealthy and unrealistic body images propagated by contemporary society. Anorexia and bulimia abound because of our inability to perceive our truest and best size and body mass. Trust God and pray for a weight loss that is divinely willed.

4. *A healthy and balanced state.* Simple weight loss does not guarantee health. For many of us, it makes a large difference, but it is not the end of the process. Health and balance involve healthy foods, a good supply of vitamins and minerals, meaningful exercise, attention to and management of stress and a growing awareness and appreciation of one's emotional and spiritual needs.

5. *Eating habits that support health and life energy.* This means we are asking God to make us conscious

eaters. Overeating is almost always a result of un-conscious eating habits. Many of us are capable of devouring entire bags of potato chips, whole gal-lons of ice cream and complete pizzas without being aware of a single bite. Awareness of the taste, smell, feel and amount of food we consume is vital to short- and long-term weight loss.

6. *Teach me to love my body.* Loving your body *before, during and after* you are overweight means loving yourself. This part of the prayer will move you to-ward an increase in self-acceptance and self-esteem, both of which are clearly God's will for your life. It is also an encouragement to treat your body with sensitivity and care. It is the only body you have, and it is time to love it even as God loves it.

If you are a participant in the Prayer Diet, it is clear that weight loss is important to you. Please remember, however, that prayer can and will bring more than a lighter body. Simply praying the Dieter's Prayer every day will connect you to your spiritual source. This con-nection can be enormously useful and transforming. It can bring insight, guidance, healing, positive change, re-lease from pain, increased self-esteem and self-love, a sense of purpose and a greatly expanded sense of the wonder of life itself.

Daily conversation with God (prayer) will change you. Often it will change you in ways you could never predict. Besides losing weight, you may discover that you are more forgiving and patient, more loving and understanding. Many report that they are more at peace and less anxious. The list of expansions, insights, healings—even miracles—is endless. The point is that something wonderful will occur. Expect it. Look for and enjoy it. Then pray some more.

> *There is a prayer that lives at the very center of your heart. If you pray it, your life will be changed forever. How does it begin?*

# Five

# MAINTAINING WEIGHT LOSS

---

"There's a moon inside every human being.
Learn to be companions with it. Give

more of your life to this listening. As
brightness is to time, so are you to

the one who talks to the deep ear in
your chest. I should sell my tongue

and buy a thousand ears when that
one steps near and begins to speak."

—Jelaludin Rumi

---

It is clear that the Prayer Diet works. People who pray the Dieter's Prayer lose weight. It is also clear that, as with any other weight-loss program, the long-term issue is how to sustain that weight loss. No one wants to lose fifty pounds, only to regain it six months later.

Maintaining weight loss requires what I call a "prayer maintenance program." We have to keep praying. Prayer must become a way of life for us, and that prayer must lead to a deeper understanding of ourselves and what drives us to overeat. This should not be difficult if prayers have already produced weight-loss results, but even the most dedicated can use support.

Weight loss is a complex and difficult journey. Even though the Prayer Diet is powerful and effective, it is not a magic bullet that will eliminate deeper energies that ultimately control eating habits. If you are affected by low self-esteem, self-hate, childhood traumas or painful emotions, you need to attend to them. If you avoid them, you will discover prayer alone is not enough and you will regain the weight you worked so hard to lose.

Here are four prayers that will help you find God's guidance and healing. They are prayers that I have used for years. They will focus your heart and mind on the unavoidable issues that control eating habits and will enable you to receive God's healing.

There is no formula for praying these prayers. You may pray them as you need them. But, sooner or later, we need them all. No one is exempt from the influence of deep psychological drives and energies. I share this truth as one who tried to ignore them and suffered enormously. Use the prayers regularly. God will do the rest.

### The Prayer for Self-Love

*Father / Mother God, you know everything my mind thinks and my heart feels. You know how mercilessly I criticize and damn myself. You know that I am often incapable of forgiving myself for mistakes and imperfections and sometimes for simply existing. You know more than anyone how I suffer from self-condemnation and self-hate.*

*Dear loving God, deliver me from the hell I create for myself. Teach me to forgive myself. Teach me to see myself through Your eyes of compassion. Show me how to love every aspect of who I have been, am now and can be.*

*Dear Divine Source, I surrender my self-condemning will to your loving and accepting will. I surrender my judgment to your compassion. And I open my heart without reservation to your tender care and nurture. Amen.*

We must pray this prayer as if our lives depended on it. Mine did and still does. My experience with self-hate was like an internal holocaust. It was out of control until I finally faced it, admitted its influence in every aspect of my life and began to pray for God's guidance.

My most powerful encounter with self-hate took place in Hawaii fifteen years ago. I decided to use a Jungian technique called active imagination and write a dialogue with my inner judge. I had written this kind of dialogue with other internal parts of myself many times before and always with great benefit. I had dreamed about this inner persecutor the night before and knew that it was time to go much deeper in my attempts to manage or heal it.

I took my notebook and drew a line down the center of the page. In the left-hand column I was going to allow my inner judge to say whatever it wanted to say. In the right-hand column I was going to write my healthier, self-loving reactions and responses. I was not prepared for what happened.

I allowed my Inner Judge to speak first and it erupted with rage and condemnation of every aspect of my life. It attacked my body, my work, my relationships and my value as a human being. It was vicious, merciless and extremely abusive. It went on and on and on until, unable to breathe, I stopped writing and put the notebook down.

When I returned to what I had written, I was shocked at what I saw. Of course I was dismayed at the intensity of the judge's rage and what that meant about the degree of self-hate, but I was more devastated by what I did not see. I had written three detailed pages of self-condemning abuse. The left-hand column was full. But the right-hand side of the three pages was blank. I had not written a single word in self-defense.

I felt I as if I had come face-to-face with a force that was almost demonic. It seemed larger than life and much more than a dream figure. If I had been living in the thirteenth or fourteenth century, I would have sworn I was a man possessed. Thanks to contemporary psychology, however, I was able to name it for what it really was . . . serious self-hate.

As I looked at the painful evidence of my self-destructive energies, I made myself a promise. I swore I would find a way to confront and ultimately heal this harmful inner force. I promised myself I would not live the second half of my life under the control of its poisonous directives.

There was no easy answer, but step by step I was led to inner healing and the ability to forgive myself, accept myself and love myself. The journey to self-love has been difficult because I have often resisted it and, on occasion, the inner judge still raises its ugly head. But God has been patient and faithful, and I have persevered.

The result has been remarkable. I no longer hate myself. I am no longer plagued with intense bouts of self-criticism or condemnation. I am capable of saying no to the Inner Judge who used to rule my self-perception. And I no longer eat to dull the pain because the pain is no longer there.

> *What if you really believed that God loves you more than you love yourself? Would you be willing to surrender your self-hate to his greater love? Will you now?*

My prayers for self-love and compassion produced wonderful results. They were answered by the timely appearance of insightful books, talented and compassionate therapists, dozens of healing and inspiring workshops and hundreds of courageous clients.

I also found concerned friends, forgiving children, a perceptive and incredibly loving wife and a mysterious and magnificent universe that nurtures my soul every minute of every day.

The more I prayed, the more I became aware of how specific and sensitive the answers were. Help arrived from every corner of my life. My car radio spoke to me every time I turned the dial. Bumper stickers on the cars around me contained useful messages. Even junk mail that I never opened would have words and phrases on the envelopes that would be healing.

I was bombarded with help and slowly began to let it in. Eventually, I shifted from self-hate to a new sense of value, self-acceptance, self-love and an almost over-whelming awareness of God's pervasive presence.

Wherever you are on this difficult journey, I invite you to pray this prayer. We need all the help we can get, and now is the time to ask for it. It will make a difference in your growth and healing.

### The Prayer for Healing Difficult Emotions

*O God, sometimes my feelings are so frightening and intense that I will do anything to make them disappear. My body seems too small to hold the powerful and confusing emotions that overwhelm me. I feel as if I am a cork thrown about by the waves of a stormy ocean. I feel powerless to manage these inner forces, and so I am praying for your help and guidance.*

*Dear God, hold me in your arms and protect me when my difficult emotions appear. Keep me safe and aware of each feeling and help me correctly interpret its valuable message. Teach me how to be with, accept and wisely manage my anger, hurt, fear, sadness and every other intense emotion that I am capable of feeling.*

*Give me, loving Guide, the courage to greet every emotion with an open mind and heart so that I can grow and heal from the lessons they bring me.*

*And finally, dear Creator, remind me that my feelings are ultimately gifts and treasures of the heart that allow me to fully experience the wonder of being human. Amen.*

I have written articles and spoken at workshops about the relationship between intense feelings and unhealthy eating habits. I call this process "eating to kill," because it is clear those of us who are overweight eat to kill our difficult emotions. Whenever a feeling we fear begins to arise, we go directly to our drug of choice . . . food. As soon as we start eating, we feel better. The uncomfortable feeling subsides because food literally changes our body chemistry and numbs the expected pain.

I am convinced that every individual who is chronically overweight (twenty-five pounds or more) is a food addict who uses food to kill uncomfortable feelings. As addicts, we are afraid of our emotions and have few management skills. We have never learned to identify, learn or heal from our intense emotions. We tend to see powerful feelings as enemies that only want to harm us. We assume we would be overwhelmed, or even destroyed, if we did not do everything in our power to stop, numb or at least lessen our strong internal reactions to life.

This kind of anachronistic logic pervades our culture a hundred years after the discovery of modern psychology. We have "demonized" our strong emotions, and any feeling that threatens to rise in intensity above "mild" faces potential exorcism by denial or by the favorite American drug . . . food.

In truth, our feelings are an essential part of what makes us human. God has given us the gift of emotion. The infinite depth of our emotional system makes it possible for us to relate intimately to our own souls and to God.

Our feelings are our protectors, guides, blessings and teachers. Their level of intensity is almost always in direct relationship to the importance of their message. How, then, can we expect to lead wise and healthy lives if we constantly kill the messenger before he has an opportunity to speak?

If we eat to kill our feelings, we will be left without a God-sent friend and teacher. How, then, can we expect to work, love, live and eat without significant problems? If we constantly ignore, repress or drug these powerful energies, how can we be surprised when they suddenly break through their internal cages and disrupt our best-laid plans for weight loss?

As I was writing this chapter, I spotted a book by Matthew Fox, *Original Blessing*. I picked it up and allowed it to fall open to a page. At the top of the page, in my own handwriting, were the words *"Do not run from your pain."*

This kind of synchronicity, as the Jungians call it, has followed many of my heartfelt prayers. The book itself had appeared to me in a rather unusual way. It "found me" at the only library book sale I have ever attended. I purchased it in 1986 for a dollar and was introduced to the provocative work of theologian Matthew Fox. I took the book home and immersed myself for two days, underlining almost every other paragraph. Since then, I have read everything Matthew Fox has written, and each book has moved me further along my spiritual path.

The notes that caught my attention were from the section entitled "Being Emptied: Letting Pain Be Pain: Kenosis." I had drawn a line from my notes to a paragraph I had underlined twice.

> *"Facing the darkness, admitting the pain, allowing the pain to be pain, is never easy. That is why courage—bigheartedness—is the most essential virtue on the spiritual journey. But if we fail to let pain be pain—and our entire patriarchal culture refuses to let this happen—then pain will haunt us in nightmarish ways . . . There is no way to let go of pain without first embracing it and loving it—not as pain but as a sister and brother . . . First comes the embrace, the allowing of pain to be pain; next comes the journey with the pain; then the letting go . . . into a cauldron where the pain's energy will serve us. And finally comes the benefit we do indeed derive from having burned this fuel."*

In a few words, Matthew Fox has brought us into and through the entire process. Pain, which most often appears as difficult emotions, must be embraced, worked through, then celebrated because of the gifts it always contains. Fox goes on to describe those five gifts. They are: compassion, the ability to understand pleasure, an increase in strength to continue the journey, a deep linking and bonding with others and a powerful uniting with the universe.

The words "Do not run from your pain" obviously hold great promise. They are not an invitation to masochism but an opportunity for deep and meaningful transformation and growth. They need to be constantly remembered as we confront the many emotions that weight loss exposes.

In order to maintain our hard-won weight loss, we must pray for God's help with our difficult emotions. Once we have prayed, we need to listen carefully to his answers and follow them closely. In many cases, this means embarking on an eventful and life-changing inner journey . . . a journey that will lead us to a more compassionate and greatly expanded vision of who we are and what we are worth.

### JANICE AND ANGER

Janice was a client who has used this prayer to achieve unusual results in her growth. She came to me to explore the deeper causes of her destructive eating patterns. After three sessions, it became obvious Janice had a problem with anger. She did not appear to be an angry person. Her friends considered her to be easygoing and even-tempered. But below the surface, Janice was angry and was terrified to express it.

Janice had grown up with a father who was a rageaholic . . . a person addicted to fits of uncontrollable rage. Janice, her siblings and her mother had been frequently abused by the father's anger binges. She had vowed never to be that way. As a result, Janice was unable to express even the slightest frustration for fear of being like Dad. She had learned to eat away her anger instead of expressing it. By the time she was forty, she was a hundred pounds overweight.

When I began to discuss this idea with Janice, she became afraid. She worried I was trying to make her like her father. Eventually she realized that anger did not have to be abusive. I explained that the solution to her anger and weight problem was not to act out the anger, but to learn to feel and be with the emotion. Then she could learn constructive ways of managing and expressing it. Once this occurred, she would not need to eat the anger away.

I constructed a version of the Prayer to Heal Difficult Emotions for Janice and asked her to pray it three or four times a day while we continued our exploration of her fear of anger. She agreed because the prayer gave her a sense of protection and safety.

After a month, Janice noticed a change in her relationship to her anger. She said she was much more aware of feeling angry and had even expressed a bit of it to a friend on two occasions. She was thrilled she was able to notice, then talk about it without hurting her friend. She told me the prayer made her feel as if God would protect her from using the anger destructively. I agreed and asked her to keep praying.

In another month, Janice said she was beginning to lose weight. It was only five pounds, but she was excited because she was not on a formal diet. We continued to work on anger, and she kept praying faithfully each day. After another six months, Janice had lost fifty pounds. At that point, she decided she could continue without my weekly support and went on her way. She contacted me about three months later to say she had lost another twenty pounds.

Janice's experience is not unique. Prayer can make a difference for all of us, and is especially helpful with frightening and painful feelings.

Like Janice, you do not need to eat to kill your feelings. You can find immediate help, healing and guidance that will liberate you from this inner prison. I invite you to start by praying the Prayer to Heal Difficult Emotions. Pray it often and expect answers. They will come, and they will make a difference.

## The Prayer for Openness and Vision

*Dear All-Seeing and All-Knowing Presence, I pray that you will make me aware of my strong attachment to my perceptions, beliefs and attitudes. Break down the walls that block*

*my vision and open my mind and heart to the unlimited
manifestations of your love and guidance and care.*

*Teach me to see with your sight, hear with your ears and feel
with your heart. Give me the courage to let go of my limited
expectations of your power and creativity. Lift me up from my
narrow and darkened hiding places and fill me with the
light of your infinite wisdom. Amen.*

Little hinders us more from seeing God's timely answers to prayers than our rigid attachment to limited beliefs and attitudes. I am reminded of the story about the
shaman who healed a woman's eyesight. After receiving a
miraculous healing and being able to see better than she
had in years, the woman asked her son if the shaman was
a Christian. Unwilling to lie to her, he told her the truth.
No, he was not a Christian, he was a Native American
healer.

The woman's belief about the legitimate scope of
healing immediately asserted itself. She believed no true
healing could come from anyone who was not a Christian. Within days, her eyes reverted to their previous
condition. The miracle was reversed.

This woman was not unique. Many of us are attached
to our version of truth and remain blind to God's loving
answers to our prayers because they do not fit our belief
systems.

The results of our selective blindness are tragic. We
pray fervent prayers. God responds specifically and lov-

ingly, yet we remain ignorant and unaware of the miracle that stands before us. With such limited vision, it is no wonder that we pray less and expect less from our relationship with God.

What might occur if you prayed for expanded vision and openness to God's special way of working in your life? What miracle, heretofore unseen and unexperienced, might appear? What might be the effect on your ability to trust, to believe and to have faith in a loving and caring God?

My mentor, Rumi, tells another ancient story that makes the point better than I can.

## THE HOLY MAN AND THE SNAKE

Once there was a holy man who made a trip across a vast desert. One afternoon he arrived at an oasis, where he saw a fellow traveler sleeping in the shade of a palm tree. The traveler was lying on his side, snoring loudly with his mouth wide open. Without warning, a poisonous snake slithered out of the grass into his mouth and down his throat.

Immediately, the holy man went into action. He shook the traveler to wake him, then began to hit him with his riding crop and ordered him to run around the oasis. The shaken traveler recognized the holy man and became frightened. Why was this man of God torturing him? As he ran, he begged for an explanation. "Sir, why are you angry at me? I have not offended you. Holy father, please tell me. What has happened? Why do you punish me so?"

Without explaining, the holy man demanded that the exhausted traveler fall on his knees and begin to eat mud by the handfuls. Terrified, the man complied and soon became so ill that he threw up the contents of his stomach, including the deadly snake.

The thankful man threw himself at the feet of the wise and compassionate holy man. "Thank you, O friend of God. By your wisdom and benevolent action, you have saved my life. From this day forth, I will be your devoted disciple."

An innocent man on a long journey goes to sleep in the peaceful shade of a palm tree. Suddenly he is awakened and apparently tortured by a man of God. Has he sinned unknowingly? Has God decided to punish him for no reason? He is hurt, frightened and confused until the source of his problem is finally revealed. Then in a single, insightful moment, everything is transformed from horror to blessing.

Much of life is like Rumi's tale. Everything depends on what we see and how we see it. Too often, we see horror when blessing is upon us. Too often we believe that momentary discomfort means something is wrong. Too often we curse life and God because we do not have the vision to see the deeper truth before us.

What would happen if you saw your weight in the light of this story? I imagine if you are anything like I used to be, you hate your excess weight. "Fat hate" is the norm for our society. To put it in terms of the story, your fat would be symbolized by the snake. You see it as something dangerous to your health. That perception would not be unusual.

But what would a change in perception do for you? What if you were able to see your weight as the holy man saw the snake? What if your excess weight was a catalyst goading you toward deeper healing, self-care, self-love, greater self-esteem, increased self-expression and a transformed relationship with life and God?

*What if God himself has sent the weight to your body, not as a punishment, but as a gift that will ultimately bless you?* If you could see clearly that this was the real truth about your excess weight, how would you feel? How would your life change?

The last of the great Roman emperors, Marcus Aurelius (A.D. 121–180), wrote an amazingly enlightened and timelessly appropriate entry in his journal, *The Meditations.* It could have been written by a contemporary spiritual teacher and certainly applies to all of us.

*"Everything is turned to one's advantage when he greets a situation like this: 'You are the very thing I was looking for.' Truly, whatever arises in life is the right material to bring about your growth and the growth of those around you. This, in a word, is art—and this art called 'life' is a practice suitable to both men and gods. Everything contains some special purpose and a hidden blessing; what then could be strange or arduous, when all of life is here to greet you like an old and trusted friend?"*

I am fully aware that I am posing a potentially outrageous idea here. You live in a society that has taught you that fat is bad and you are bad for being fat. You have suffered from that perception. Other people's negative attitudes about fat have hurt you, but the greatest harm has been done by your own perception and belief about yourself.

If you are like the rest of the fat-haters of America, you see being overweight as a sign of weakness, lack of self-discipline and low self-esteem. To put it in common, everyday language . . . you think being fat stinks! You would get a lot of agreement on that opinion, but where does that take you? It takes you straight back to self-hate.

If you allow your perception and interpretation of excess weight to be dominated by the foolish minds of fat haters, you will never see its amazing and life-transforming gifts. If you continue to hold tightly to the popular view of fat, you will remain blind to God's work and purpose in your life.

## JACK'S STORY

Jack was thirty-two years old, five-feet-six and seventy-five pounds overweight when he first walked into my office. He had been heavy since childhood. His life had been marked with memories of shame and ridicule by other kids who called him names and showed no mercy or sensitivity. As a result, Jack hated his body and made no distinction between his physical identity and his personal worth. Jack hated Jack, and he blamed his fat for everything.

Jack told me he would do anything to change his body. He had reached the end of his emotional rope and felt desperate. He was thirty-two and had never had a lover or a meaningful relationship. He was convinced his weight was the reason. As he spoke, he wept tears of frustration and despair. He completed his story with a question: "Is there any hope for me?"

My first comments seemed to shock him, but he listened carefully. I told him the answer to his question was up to him. I said hope was possible, but only if he was willing to let go of something he had learned to cherish and value more than anything else in his life: His hate for his fat.

Jack's response was anger. He was insulted that I would tell him he cherished the very thing that had caused his suffering. I told him I fully understood his anger, but his way of dealing with fat had never worked and hope would only appear if he tried something new. He stopped talking, took a breath and said, "O.K., you are right about that. Please explain yourself so I don't have to walk out of here right now."

Jack and I then began a dialogue that would last for months. First, I introduced him to the idea of "mental blindness," then the power of prayer. I asked him to pray for openness of mind every day and to try to be open to the messages God would bring him as a result of his requests. Jack thought this was rather silly, but he agreed to follow my directions.

Over the next six months, Jack experienced a breakthrough. He underwent a significant change in his relationship to his body and, more importantly, to himself and to God. He began to see that his body weight had nothing to do with his personal value or his ability to relate to people, especially women. He also learned to listen, without anger, to the lessons his excess weight had to teach him.

Jack discovered that his eating habits were related to deeper issues, and those issues were the real causes of his pain and unhappiness. He eventually began to date a young woman and enthusiastically announced to me that she did not care about his body size.

We worked together for over a year, and Jack found hope, a new sense of worth and changed his ability to see himself and his weight. We gave most of the credit to his constant prayer for openness. Jack often told me he could almost feel his mind stretch and his eyes open to see things differently. We both believe he experienced a miracle.

You are no different from Jack. If you pause for a moment to consider his story, you will see you are being offered a new vision of your weight and of God's presence in your life. God has ways of working that may initially seem confusing, but are ultimately miraculous. The very thing you experience as a major source of pain can become a source of joy. To become aware of this truth requires a shift in vision. That shift can occur through prayer.

Don't take my word or Jack's for this. You only have

to pray the Prayer for Openness and Vision. God will do the rest. When your ability to see through his eyes occurs, you will have a rush of renewed faith, peace and a sense of belonging that you may never have known before.

## The Prayer of Total Surrender

*"Thy will be done"* is the simplest, but most powerful, of all prayers. There is no other prayer that means more, implies more or accomplishes more. In four short, uncomplicated words, this prayer says more than all other prayers combined. In fact, it is so significant and potentially transforming that it should not be prayed by the spiritual beginner.

*"Thy will be done"* is the prayer to pray after we completely and totally fall in love with God. It is the prayer of a lover so filled with passion for his beloved that he has no more room for himself in his body. He cries out, as Rumi did, *"I am a wine-glass, you are granite. Guess what happens when we meet."*

*"Thy will be done"* is a prayer that emerges naturally from a heart that has come to know the ultimate trustability and care of God. It rises spontaneously from a heart that has been so frequently comforted and healed by divine nurture that it has nothing else to ask for.

*"Thy will be done"* is a prayer that has no "I" in it. The individual has no reason to be. Only complete immersion in divine will can suffice.

*"Thy will be done"* is a prayer of total surrender. When

we pray this prayer, we no longer include our specific wishes, needs or desires. We give up our attempts to control or direct God's behavior. We admit and accept that our vision is limited, and we entrust our well-being to God's care.

This prayer may be particularly difficult to pray when we are desperate about losing weight. We have a very specific need, and we usually have a clear idea of how many pounds we want to lose. We want to say, *"Dear God, please help me lose forty-five pounds."* We want to control our weight destiny because we are so convinced that losing weight is the right thing to do and we are often exactly right.

I am not invalidating the Dieter's Prayer here. I encourage you to pray that prayer regularly and to expect to lose weight. I am also saying that eventually you will come to experience God's divine wisdom so completely, you will need no other prayer.

### The Power of Nondirect Prayer

In his book *Healing Words,* Dr. Larry Dossey describes a study about the effects of something he calls "nondirect prayer" or "the thy will be done approach." He cites studies that not only provide scientific proof that prayer works but also indicate nondirect prayer produces better results than directed prayer!

Directed prayer is described as prayer that "has a specific goal, image or outcome in mind. Those who pray are 'directing' the system (God), attempting to steer it in a precise direction." He then goes on to make the following rather amazing comments.

> *"Which prayer technique—directed or nondirected—is more effective? It is important to bear in mind that the* most important discovery is that prayer works and that both methods are effective. *But in the tests, the nondirected technique appeared quantitatively more effective, frequently yielding results that were twice as great, or more, when compared to the directed approach . . . On the basis of a large number of tests, when a nondirected prayer is answered, the outcome is always in the direction of 'what's best for the organism.'"*

Dr. Dossey has scientifically confirmed a fact about nondirected, "thy will be done" prayer that mystics and other experienced devotees of all religions have known for millennia. If we translate this fact to spiritual language, we might say, *"God has a better vision of what is best for us than we do. Trusting in God's will rather than our own always produces the best outcome."*

I suggest you pray this prayer when you are ready and not before. Begin your weight-loss prayers with the Dieter's Prayer, then slowly add the other prayers I have included. After you have assured yourself that prayer works and God specifically cares about you, begin to add "thy will be done" to your prayers. Remember, God listens more to the cries of your heart than your words. He knows what you need. Open your mind and heart to receive it.

## More About Weight Loss, Prayer and Surrender

Americans are obsessed with control. We spend billions of dollars annually on books, CDs, workshops and success gurus to teach us how to lose weight, create our own destinies and increase the size of our portfolios. For the first fifty years of my life, I was a card-carrying control freak. I was certain I was the author of my future. I was convinced the achievements and successes I desired would be mine if I took responsibility, set clear goals and worked the principles the gurus of achievement prescribed.

On occasion, I proved them right. Sometimes I envisioned a goal, laid out a plan for achieving it, worked the plan with commitment and arrived at exactly the place I said I wanted to be. A few times, I even exceeded my expectations. The experience was heady and empowering, and I began to assume I had the magic formula for controlling my destiny. I was naive, and I was mistaken. Eventually, life taught me an important lesson: Control is an illusion.

You are reading this book because you want to lose weight. I have told you that praying will cause you to lose that weight. It may seem that, like the gurus of success, I am giving you a technique to control your weight and even to control God. I am not.

Prayer, especially the Dieter's Prayer, is a call for help. It is an admission of powerlessness. It is an acknowledgment of our inability to control our eating patterns and, ultimately, our own bodies. Prayer is our way of telling

God we can't do this by ourselves and we need Her to take over.

Every addict who ever enters a twelve-step program discovers this painful but ultimately healing reality. The first step requires us to admit we are powerless over the addiction. We cannot progress to the other eleven steps and to recovery until we make this admission. This requirement is such a mental and emotional roadblock to many addicts that they remain stuck at this step for months or years. The idea of being out of control is more abhorrent than the devastating effects of their addiction.

I have compassion for these control junkies. Before I experienced the wonder of surrender, I thought being in charge of my own destiny was better than any drug. I did not realize that my personal power and control over my life had significant limitations. I understand any individual's resistance to the idea and reality of powerlessness. It is scary, confusing and initially humiliating. No normal person accepts this truth without a fight. I was one of the normal ones.

The day we look in the mirror and realize we are fat is the day we begin the journey toward surrender. But we don't arrive there overnight. First we must explore the surprising inadequacies of willpower and self-discipline. They work for a while, but that while always ends and we are fat again. We look frantically for a diet or exercise technique that will put us "back in charge of our bodies," and once again we are hopeful we can "make it happen." Pretty soon we are fat again.

Eventually, after dozens of failed diet and exercise

programs, many of us become hopeless. It is this painful, but unavoidable, encounter with hopelessness that becomes the vehicle for a breakthrough that can change us forever. We finally admit we are out of control and need help in a way and at a level we have never experienced before. Now we are ready to pray.

Prayer for weight loss is a prayer of surrender. We are admitting to ourselves and to God that this is outside the limits of our power. We are admitting that our food consumption, our food choices, our binges and all our self-destructive eating patterns are bigger than our willpower and self-discipline. We are saying, "Help, help, help, help." And our journey to surrender has progressed enormously.

### SURRENDER: A PERSONAL EXAMPLE

I have often been an "anxious eater." I ate when I felt anxious, and I was frequently anxious. Such foods as vegetables and fruits were useless as anxiety reducers. Over the years, I found that bread, pasta, pizza and pie worked well. They also worked well as fat producers. Eventually, I realized that losing weight would require me to lose my anxiety. So I set out to find a workable solution.

I strongly believed in the value of psychotherapy. Almost everyone I've met could benefit enormously from three to five years of a once-a-week, one-on-one consultation with a compassionate counselor. In fact, I am of the opinion that people who have been to therapy for an extended amount of time have a definite advantage (in terms of life skills, relationships and self-awareness) over those who have not. I have spent the better part of twelve years, over a twenty-five-year time span, in counseling, and I value every minute. But my anxiety was immune to it.

I progressed and grew and changed in a hundred other important and productive ways, but I still felt anxious almost every day and hated it. Psychotherapy was a "God-send" to me, but I never made one ounce of progress with my anxiety until I learned about the prayer of surrender.

I related the story about the dream I had when I was fifty. Soon after, I began the journey into the anxiety-relieving territory of surrender. I began to pray the prayer "Thy will be done" more often, and something in my mind and heart began to change. That change has almost entirely eliminated my anxiety.

I realized, through the effects of the prayer, that my anxiety had two sources. One was my predilection for living in the future. I had a habit of projecting myself forward to prepare for events and situations I felt would be difficult. It was a way of trying to protect myself against "bad" results and, ultimately, was an attempt to control life itself. This habitual future-projecting was a major source of anxiety because it never worked. The future is not real and cannot be controlled, and the more I attempted to fix, manipulate and control it, the more anxious I felt.

The second source of my anxiety was my attitude toward God. I did not trust God to take care of me. I believed in God's unconditional love and care, but I imagined he would, every once in a while, let me down. I know that this sounds irrational, but irrationality is a common aspect of theology. I believed God loved me but wasn't sure if I could always count on him. That made me anxious. If I asked God to take over completely, I might get screwed. I can't say it more honestly and clearly than that.

But I was aware I had little choice, given my position in life: "What works in the first half of life will not work in the second" (C.G. Jung). So I kept on praying "Thy will be done," over and over. After a while, the usual miracle began to manifest. I became less anxious. I found my thinking about God's trustability was shifting. I discovered spiritual synchronicity was leading me to books and people and experiences that supported my faith in the ultimate love and care of God.

I began to feel relieved that I did not have to control everything and everyone. I felt a growing peacefulness that was better than the absence of anxiety. Most of all, I began to fall in love with God at a level I had never experienced. The prayer had introduced me to God in a way that provoked spontaneous affection and appreciation for his attention and guidance. I had found the antidote to my anxiety: *Thy will be done.*

### Prayer, Forgiveness and Weight Loss

Too often, the emotional weight of the past becomes the physical weight of the present. Think back on your life and remember someone who hurt you. Picture that individual and ask this question. "Have I forgiven that person?" My guess, given that he or she appeared at this moment, is no. You have not forgiven them.

Next question. "Do you want to forgive that person?" Before you answer, consider this. The pain that person caused you has not gone away if you have not forgiven them. It remains with the memory. It does not matter if you try to forget the event or rarely even think about it.

The pain remains, and that pain affects you every single day. It is an emotional weight that may often contribute to your physical weight problem. I wish we could simply forget the painful past and allow it to disappear, but we cannot. Whether we like it or not, we do not find release from our past until we face it and, most often, forgive it.

Let's go back to the person who hurt you. What kind of feelings arise as you think about them? What memories surround the feelings? The pain that begins to emerge is the pain that remains. That pain lives day to day in your heart and in your "gut." The question to ask is, "Do I want to continue to live with this pain?"

I assume the answer to the last question is no, you do not want to live with this pain. But if you are like many of us, you believe you have no choice. You think the past cannot be changed and the pain cannot be removed. Thank God, you are mistaken.

Forgiveness can remove the pain of the past. It will not remove the memory, but it will erase the hurt, anger and humiliation and the other painful emotions that accompanied it. Once you learn to forgive, you will be freed from the weight the hurt created in your heart. Forgiveness will release you from the toxic bonds of your painful past. It is a way out of the dark emotional woods that surround you.

Many of us resist forgiveness because we think it means we are letting the other person off the hook. We believe forgiveness is a way of making the painful event insignificant. Nothing could be further from the truth. If the event were truly insignificant, we would not need to forgive. Forgiveness is only appropriate when something significant has occurred. If you were raped when you were ten, that is terribly significant. That event has had a major effect on your life. To consider forgiving the rapist does not mean you are making light of the rape and its damage to your body, your mind and your sense of self. Instead, forgiveness is a way of confirming the power of the event and offering you a way to finally put it behind you. Forgiveness will release you from the trauma, once and for all.

Forgiveness will not work until you understand this point: It provides you with a way out of the pain. When you clearly realize this, you will welcome forgiveness the way a starving man welcomes a piece of bread. It will heal your hurt and allow you to drop the emotional weight of the past. Once you forgive, you will actually feel lighter and happier, more at peace and more alive.

> *What if God actually loves to forgive? What if God is overjoyed at the prospect of helping you learn forgiveness? What prayer would you pray then?*

## FORGIVING OTHERS—A SIMPLE EXERCISE

Find a quiet room or space outdoors. Sit down and take a few deep breaths. Then begin your forgiveness session with a prayer. You may create your own prayer, but I have included the one I often use. I am convinced prayer is an essential part of the forgiveness process because we need God's help to open our hearts to the person who harmed us. Here is my prayer. You may want to read it aloud when you do this exercise.

> *"Dear Forgiving Friend, I want to learn to forgive and I need your help. Please take away my anger, my hurt, my disappointment and all my painful feelings related to this person. Give me the strength to forgive and to let go of this painful event in my past. Amen."*

Once you have prayed the prayer, close your eyes and imagine the person you are going to forgive is sitting in front of you. It is your fantasy, so place that person in a chair and make him quiet and receptive to what you have to say. Then proceed to the next step.

Tell that person clearly and directly what he did to harm you. Tell him how it has affected you, your life, your relationships and your sense of self. Tell him how you have felt about him. Then tell him that you have suffered enough and are ready to let go of your pain. From this day you want to go forward without the pain they caused.

Tell the person that with God's help, you forgive him.

*"I forgive you with all my heart and soul and with the help of God. I forgive you for every act and word and thought that brought me pain. I forgive you, and I release you from my past. I forgive you, and I bless you, and I send you on your way. Go in peace as I go my own way in peace."*

Imagine you stand up, turn around and walk away into your own peaceful future. Don't look back. Keep walking until you get to a beautiful mountain or lake or ocean. Then stand at the water or on the mountain and thank God for forgiveness. Pray a prayer of thanks for the wonderful power that has released you from the pain and hurt of your past. Then go into the present at peace.

Note: Remember, the memory of the event that harmed you will not disappear. When it returns, simply bless it and remind yourself you forgave and let it go. As time goes on, this will occur less and less.

If you want to have a dramatic experience of losing emotional weight that will almost always affect your destructive eating patterns, try this. Make a list of every person who has ever hurt you since you were born. Write them all down. You may be surprised at the number of names, but don't allow that to stop you. I did this exercise about ten years ago, and I had eighty-six names by the time I stopped writing. I was shocked, but I was also happy I could do something productive with all that emotional baggage.

Once you have the list, start at the top and work your way down. Use the exercise above and forgive every single one of these people, whether they are dead or alive. Do not ask if they deserve to be forgiven. Deserving is not the issue, forgiveness is. Don't forget to begin every forgiveness session with a prayer. This kind of psychological and spiritual work cannot be done effectively without divine help. But also remember God loves to forgive and will always be a full partner with you in all forgiveness projects. Now the hard part.

## FORGIVING YOURSELF—A NOT SO SIMPLE EXERCISE

If you are like most of us, you find it easier to forgive others than yourself. However, forgiveness goes both ways or not at all. We must learn to forgive ourselves or we will have a hard time forgiving others. In truth, the person in our lives in greatest need of forgiveness is us. If you will look honestly at your deepest thoughts, you will see you are the person you judge the most. If you really want to let go of a giant load of emotional baggage, you will have to learn to forgive yourself. How about starting today? Let's start with a prayer.

*"Merciful and gracious God:*

*Now I need more help than ever. I need to learn to forgive myself. I am sure that I cannot do this by myself. I am full of self-judgment and self-recrimination, and I am certain that my judgments are right. Please fill me with your love and mercy. Give me your gift of forgiveness and show me how to forgive myself. Amen."*

If you are like me, you will want to pray this prayer eight or nine times just to warm up. Forgiving yourself is difficult, and I am sure many of you have, until now, found it impossible. I am convinced much of the physical weight obese people carry is due to their inability to forgive themselves. We are often driven by an irrational inner voice that expects perfection and never cuts us any slack. Forgiveness is out of the question to this merciless judge.

The tragedy is without the ability to forgive ourselves, we increase our emotional baggage on a daily basis. Every day we make mistakes, and every day we condemn ourselves for them. No wonder we eat so much. Food is often the only drug available to ease the pain. The trouble is, every day the weight, both emotional and physical, gets heavier. No diet in the world is ever going to overcome these powerful forces unless we learn to forgive. And that includes forgiving ourselves.

So, pray the prayer again and do the following exercise. I have made it a regular part of my weekly routine and it makes an enlightening difference.

Make a list similar to the first list above, except this time make it about your mistakes. Some people want to call these mistakes sins. If that word works for you then use it but remember this. The Christian word for sin is from the koine Greek "himartia". It is used frequently in the New Testament. Interestingly, it is a word used by archers and means "missing the mark", as when an arrow misses its target. I have used the word mistake because I am convinced that it is closest to the original meaning in Christian scripture.

The list may be a long one. Be sure to include everything that comes to mind, whether it makes sense or not. Once you have the completed list, start at the top and work your way down. This may take quite awhile. You may want to do an hour a day for a week or two instead of trying a forgiveness marathon. Take your time. It is worth every ounce of effort.

Pick item No. 1, pray the prayer and do the following. Imagine yourself sitting in a chair in a quiet room. Then imagine that you are entering the room and sitting in front of the other you. When you are ready, talk about the mistake. Describe it in detail. Describe how it affected you and anyone else involved. Also describe how this mistake has made you feel about yourself.

Now begin the forgiveness part. Look directly at the you who made the mistake and say the following.

*"By the power that God so graciously has given me, I forgive you. I forgive you. I forgive you for each and every aspect of this mistake you have made. God forgives you, and I forgive*

*you. You can let go of all pain connected to this event. You are free now to live without the burden of self-judgment. I forgive you. Go in peace."*

Then imagine yourself standing up and hugging *the you that is forgiven.* Hug as long as you want, then walk out of the forgiveness room together. Do this process over and over until you have forgiven even the smallest mistakes. By the time you get to the middle of the list, you will have developed a lifelong ability to forgive yourself.

Each forgiveness will make you lighter in heart and mind and body. Eventually, everyone around you will notice a difference in your attitude about life. You have nothing to lose but your pain.

> *What if forgiveness could become as easy as prayer? What if forgiveness was as natural as breathing? Who and what would you forgive first?*

## Last Words About Maintaining Weight Loss

To conclude this chapter, I want to give you my best advice about sustaining weight loss. If you have been a chronically overweight person, you will have to be weight-sensitive for the rest of your life. I think this is a good thing. It is good because it requires you to pay constant attention to prayer, inner work and your relationship with God.

As I said above, I see excess weight as a gift. It is a

clear and obvious sign that points us in the direction of self and God awareness. No other goal in life could have more reward than that. Sustaining weight loss, then, is an ongoing, lifelong process of inner work and prayer. Nothing can take its place, and nothing can bring us more joy.

If you have been chronically overweight, you can give thanks, because your body will always tell you when you have returned to your old, self-destructive habits. It will begin to push out its boundaries and tighten your waistband. It will persist until you have no choice but to pay attention. It will be like a trusted friend who tells you things that no one else would dare say. *"Hey, buddy, you have gotten lost for a moment. Stop and remember who you are and what you have learned."*

If you want to maintain your weight loss, I suggest you follow this simple plan.

1. Decide that God is your friend and he uses weight gain as a way of reminding you to take better care of yourself.
2. Make the Dieter's Prayer a regular part of your daily routine.
3. Pray the Prayer for Self-Love, the Prayer for Healing Difficult Emotions and the Prayer for Openness and Vision until you see dramatic progress in all three areas.
4. Then, after you have experienced God's consistent love and care so thoroughly that your heart is

bursting with joy, begin to pray *"Thy will be done"* at all times.

5. Assume your excess weight has appeared for a "special purpose" and contains a "hidden blessing" and allow God to reveal both to you in His own time.

---

*What if everything that occurs in your life is there for a purpose? What if you lived as if this was true? How would you pray, and what would you pray for?*

---

## Six

# THE AMAZING POWER
# OF PRAYER

---

*"Muhammad says,*
*'I come before dawn*
*to chain you and drag you off.'*
*It's amazing, and funny, that you have to be pulled away*
*from being tortured, pulled out*
*into this spring garden,*
*but that's the way it is.*

*Almost everyone must be bound and dragged here.*
*Only a few come on their own."*

—Jelaludin Rumi

---

Prayer is usually as communication with God. While this is true, I believe prayer is something more basic and natural. It is as essential to us as breathing. We are born with the ability to pray and it arises from our spiritual hearts as easily as blood flows from its physical counterpart. If we attempt to constrict or stop its natural movement towards God, we suffer. My term for this painful and ultimately serious condition is "spiritual deprivation". I will explore this concept and its effect on our bodies and eating patterns in a later chapter.

If we develop our natural prayer ability, we will prosper on every level that is basic to our well-being: mental, emotional, physical and spiritual. Prayer is a bridge that closes the gap between us and our Source and enables a relationship that transforms our experience of self and of God.

Most often, we think of prayer as a request for God to intervene in our daily lives. We want God to do something for us, generally as soon as possible. But there is a second aspect to prayer that is equally, if not more, important. Prayer changes the one who prays.

Prayer is an opening. Just as we must open a door to leave our house, we must open our heart to emit a prayer. Heart prayer implies that one's heart has opened to something new, something that will change the status quo of the person's interior life.

Prayer is an admission of need. We pray when we cannot control life, when we believe things are not going well. We want Divine intervention.

Prayer is an expression of gratitude. We pray when

our hearts are full of thankfulness for the wonder and awe that life brings.

Prayer is an utterance of love. We pray when we are filled with the highest and most satisfying love that exists, our love of God.

Prayer has two basic parts: sending and receiving.

> *What if one prayer could change your mind, two could change your heart and three could change your life? When would you stop praying?*

The most recognizable part of prayer is the sending. We think or speak it to God. It is formulated in our minds and hearts, then we push an internal button and it goes, like e-mail, to God's ear. For many of us, that's the end of the experience. But there is a danger in leaving out the second part . . . the receiving. We run the risk of not hearing, seeing or experiencing the answer.

I make these statements based on my firm belief that all prayer receives an answer. Therefore, the problem is not whether the prayer is answered but whether we notice that answer. We are often not open to receiving, so we imagine God has not heard us or, worse, He does not care.

Nothing blocks our willingness to pray more than a belief that God is not interested in our well-being. Nothing could be further from the truth. But this attitude is almost impossible for the unfortunate soul who cannot see results of his prayer. The answer to this blockage is receiving.

I have discovered my willingness to receive is controlled by my expectations. I often had an image of what an answered prayer should look like. If the answer did not arrive in my preconceived package, I missed it completely. I was well into my mid-thirties before I realized this significant limitation.

Once I became aware of it, my prayer life changed enormously. I had prayed intermittently, then I began to pray constantly when I discovered my perception was the problem, not God's refusal to answer.

The greatest limitation in our relationship to God is our rigid and preconceived concept of who God is. By definition, God is unknowable, yet we are persistent in our attachment to fixed images of him. This tendency is the reason for the First Commandment—*Thou shalt have no other gods before me.*

We always seem to construct limited images of God's love, abilities, wisdom, knowledge, potential and compassion. All are less than who God is. As Westerners, we could benefit greatly from a huge dose of Taoism, an ancient Chinese belief system that has wonderful teachings about this problem.

Even the most elementary Taoist knows that *"Once one speaks the Tao, that is not it."* The Divine is essentially ineffable and indefinable. Any attempt to construct limited parameters for it results in a loss of relationship. We become modern idol worshipers, focused on the idea rather than the presence itself.

If we want to pray with confidence, we need to release our preconceptions about how the answer will appear. We must open our hearts and minds to the insightful guidance God brings. This is true for any prayer, be it for healing, guidance or weight loss. We must learn to trust the greater wisdom of he who knows what is best.

Once we reach this important step in the prayer process, we can pray with great confidence that we are heard, understood and loved. Then every aspect of our lives is prayable, including issues of weight loss, eating habits, bingeing, anorexia, body image and self-esteem.

### What Can Prayer Do?

Here's the short answer: Anything and everything.

Prayer has been known to heal every illness imaginable. It has changed the weather and stopped wild animals and human beings from vicious acts. It has removed tumors, blood clots, viruses and even cavities from teeth. It has released thousands of individuals from the death grip of addiction and has enabled many to experience significant weight loss.

Since moving to Florida, I have developed a close relationship with two surgeons. Their personalities are as different as two men of the same profession could be. One is quiet, reserved and a traditional Christian. The other is outspoken, often aggressive and an enthusiastic explorer of non-traditional spiritual and medical paths. Both have been practicing for about twenty years and have significant experience with illness and its effect on the body. As I grew to know these men, it became obvious they were clearly committed to medicine. Both are highly respected by patients and the medical community.

We have had many conversations about the subjects of prayer medicine and healing. They are in total agreement about one thing . . . prayer can make a miraculous difference in the practice of medicine. Here is a story one of the doctors told me.

A patient was diagnosed with a large brain tumor. The tumor was life-threatening and possibly not operable, but a date for surgery was set. The patient told her doctor she belonged to a prayer group and they would pray about her condition.

The day before the surgery, the woman was examined again and the tumor could not be found. It had totally disappeared. The woman gave credit to prayer. The doctor had no explanation.

My physician friends tell me that stories like this are common to every area of medicine. Every physician has his prayer story with miraculous results.

As an individual who has grown up in a culture of prayer, I have no problem believing the veracity of the tumor story. I have so much experience with the power of prayer in my own life I have no doubt about its effects on the lives of others.

If you want more scientific validations of the power of prayer, I suggest you read Dr. Larry Dossey's *HEALING WORDS: The power of prayer and the practice of medicine*. Dr. Dossey has written a number of books in which he explores prayer as a scientifically observable phenomenon.

He cites cases, research and studies that should satisfy most inquiring minds.

Research into the power of prayer can be found in Deepak Chopra's book *How to Know God*. It includes prayer groups from different religions. Here is an example:

> *"In 1998, a Duke University research team verified to all skeptics that prayer, indeed, had such power. The researchers took into account all manner of variables, including heart rate, blood pressure, and clinical outcomes; 150 patients who had undergone invasive cardiac procedures were studied, but none of them knew they were being prayed for.*
>
> *"Seven religious groups around the world were asked to pray. These included Buddhists in Nepal, Carmelite nuns in Baltimore, and Virtual Jerusalem, an organization that grants e-mail requests for prayers to be written down and inserted into the Wailing Wall.*
>
> *"Researchers found that surgical patients' recovery could be from 50 to 100 percent better if someone prayed for them."*

(The Duke project, formally known as the Monitoring and Actualization of Noetic Training, presented its findings in the fall of 1998 to the American Heart Association.)

These references to prayer research are wonderful confirmations of the observable power of prayer, but they cannot compare to personal experience. Nothing is more convincing than an answer to one's own prayer. Therefore, I refer to my own experience as my best prayer authority. I am not just referring to my initial "pregnancy panic" I related earlier. I pray about almost everything and have done so for years. Therefore, I can give credit to hundreds of events and results in my life and the lives of those I have prayed for. Here are two examples.

In 1981, my family and I moved to a small basement-like apartment in San Diego. My wife and I had left a very successful situation in Boston and tried to start a counseling practice in Los Angeles the year before. We failed miserably. We were completely broke, humiliated and lost. A stranger (an answer to prayer) had offered us a small but cheap place to stay (also an answer to prayer) while we got back on our feet.

Every day was a financial horror. Every moment was filled with anxiety about money. I prayed about it all the time. *"God, please help us to find work and clients and money."*

Finally, I had to sell the Cadillac Eldorado we had bought in Boston, and I purchased a run-down and ancient Fiat sedan. It was rusty and dirty, but it was cheap.

After two weeks, I decided to make an effort to clean up the car. I washed and waxed it as best I could, then started on the interior. When I pulled up the dilapidated floor mat on the driver's side, I discovered four one hundred—dollar bills. They were folded and so old I was afraid they would disintegrate before I could get to the bank.

It was the answer to my prayer. The four hundred dollars covered a month's rent and still left some money for food. I was in tears when I showed the money to my wife. We both knew our prayers were being heard and answered.

The second example occurred when I was twenty-nine and finishing my doctoral degree. I was scheduled to have an oral examination on a Tuesday morning. I felt prepared and prayed for God to help me through the experience so I could graduate at the end of the next month. I walked into the meeting with three professors with the confidence that God was present. Then they dropped the bomb.

My advising professor announced the oral exam could not proceed because my doctoral project was unacceptable and would have to be done over. That would take at least a year.

My reaction was so intense that I have a difficult time describing it. My breathing stopped. My mind went into shock. Then I was hurt, disappointed, confused and extremely angry. I wanted to kill all three of those men, especially my adviser, who I felt had betrayed me. I was unable to talk intelligently and mumbled something in response to their devastating news as I left the room. I was so enraged that it took three months to return to the seminary grounds to make plans for the new project.

Was my prayer answered? Of course it was, but obviously not in the way I had hoped. It was answered at a level higher. I was being led into a new, life-shaping spiritual lesson, and the canceled oral exam was the catalyst. It took me five years to get the many complex lessons, but I finally understood and the experience was worth every ounce of pain.

Every prayer is answered. Sometimes the answer is exactly what we want. These types of answers are easy to observe and trust. If I need money and find it under the floor mat in my car, I have no trouble acknowledging the efficacy of prayer. Sometimes, however, the answer is not so obvious. Then I must work to understand, and that process may take years. Either way, prayer works.

Authority is an elusive thing in our culture. We trust almost no one. I give my generation, the 60s reformists, credit for this painful but necessary growth stage. We confronted authority at every level and were successful in cracking the blind trust our society had for designated authority.

The downside of this process is that many of us do not know who to trust about anything. We flounder, vacillate and wander aimlessly in search of guidance. Then, if we are not careful, we become unwitting subjects of the line Don Henley sings in the Eagles' song "Learn to Be Still." We "wind up following the wrong gods home."

When it comes to trusting prayer, we desperately need an authority that will help. Given that I am trained and ordained as a Christian minister, you would probably expect me to quote the Bible at this point. It would certainly make sense, and I would have no trouble listing hundreds of passages that could support my position. But that would do no good. It would be like preaching to the choir.

Bible quoting only persuades those who already believe, and it usually offends those who don't. I am amazed that more devoutly religious individuals are not aware of this rather obvious fact. So I am offering a more effective source of authority for you to consider . . . your own experience.

You don't have to trust me about the power of prayer. Trust your own experience. I am saying that prayer can affect every area of your life. I am saying that prayer can help you lose weight. I am not asking you to trust me. I am asking you to trust yourself and your own ability to see that the prayers that you pray produce observable results in your body and your life.

I have no doubt about this because I have seen that prayer has made a real and true difference in every aspect of my existence. That information, however, may be a "so what" to you. If you really want to know what prayer can do for you, you must pray. Then you must open your mind and heart to receive the answers. You will be convinced by seeing for yourself. Nothing is better than personal experience.

---

*What if the only limit to the power of prayer were your own most treasured expectations? Would you sacrifice them for something greater but unknown?*

---

In the case of the Prayer Diet, you need to pray specifically for weight loss. No one can argue with a scale. To illustrate the point, here is a sample of the many e-mails I have received.

*"Dear Doctor Anderson, I am so excited that I wanted to write and share some of my joy with you. I am one of those*

doubters who read your article about praying for weight loss and thought, at first, that this was a really stupid idea. I have always believed in God and in prayer, but I never thought that praying to lose weight was O.K. I think I thought prayer should be saved for bigger and more important things.

Anyway, I read the article, and for days I could not get it off my mind. Then, to shorten the story, I realized I had to try it. The truth is nothing else has ever worked for me. No other diet, that is. I got down on my knees (this is hard to admit), and I prayed that God would help me with my weight even if it was not a really big deal. I felt so relieved I couldn't believe it.

Then I made a copy of your prayer from the article, and I began to carry it around with me everywhere I went. I was afraid it wouldn't work by just praying it three times a day, so I prayed it every time I thought about it. Maybe this is a sign of little faith, but that is what I felt I had to do.

Right from the start, I began to change my feelings about food. My usual food panic began to go away. I can't tell you how much help this has been. I have been a food panic eater for most of my life. Every time I felt the panic begin, I read the prayer, sometimes three or four times, and I always felt better. Then, after praying, I did not have to gorge myself with food to make the panic go away. Thank God!

I know that you know what happened next. I lost weight. I have lost fifteen pounds over the last six weeks, and it has all *been because of prayer. I could go on and on about the other great changes this praying has caused, but this is enough for today. Thank you. You are in my prayers also."*

## Does God Really Care About My Weight Loss?

*"Is God really interested in my weight loss?"*
*"Can I ask God to help me lose weight?"*

These are the two most frequently asked questions that I receive about prayer and weight loss. Both imply a similar assumption about the nature of God. Is God the kind of God who cares about body and physical size? Who is this God who receives the prayers of the weight-loss community, and what is he really like?

Everyone who prays has a concept of God. After thirty years of conversations with friends, clients and workshop participants, I have observed that what we believe about God directly affects our willingness and ability to pray. It also darkens or enlightens our ability to see and understand his answers. I believe that one's concept of God is crucial to the prayer process. It needs specific attention to make the whole process work.

I once created a statement that I frequently write on the board in my counseling office. To me, it makes all the difference.

*If you do not love God,*
*it is simply because*
*you have not been properly introduced.*

Sadly, many of us have had a negative and often dysfunctional introduction to the Author of the Universe and Unconditional Lover of our Souls. Western society has been plagued for centuries by misguided Christian theologians and clergy more dominated by their neurotic psychology than by their experience of a loving and incredibly compassionate God.

They have introduced us to a God who is angry, jealous, critical, judgmental, capricious, often insensitive and unforgiving. He is portrayed as one who is ultimately more interested in who will be damned than saved. They have made fear the major reason we should be in a relationship with this frightening father figure. Their theology and instruction is fraught with rules, morality, lists of sins, punishments and carefully designed dogma that define who is in and who is out.

My hostility and regret about this American tragedy is evident. But I am only one of millions who have been victimized by this cynical attitude about God. It has taken me years to recover from its harmful effects and be liberated enough to become passionately in love with Him. This has been the best answer to prayer I've received.

If you have been wounded by this neurotic and fear-based aspect of traditional American religion, you now know you may be led from this forest of mistrust. *You cannot help but love God if you are properly introduced.*

---

*What if your image of God is not God himself? What if God is vastly more giving and loving than you have ever imagined? Would praying to this new God be a good idea?*

---

Let's start with one of the oldest and best stories that Jesus told. It is usually called the parable of the Prodigal Son, but that title misses the point. The title that sheds light on the true nature of God is the parable of the loving father.

A young man approaches his father and asks for his inheritance. This was unheard of since an inheritance came only after the death of the parent. Even though he was assaulted by his son's insensitive request, the father had an amazing answer. He said yes.

The son goes to another country and squanders the money. Today, we would say he spent it on sex, drugs and rock and roll. When his situation could not get worse, he does what E.T. would do . . . calls home. He decides even the servants in his father's house are better off then he, so he starts the long journey back to the home he willfully abandoned.

At this point, Jesus inserts his transforming insight into the nature of God. He tells us something almost revolutionary and certainly endearing about the father. He says the father saw the son coming home and *ran down the road to meet him*.

If you have heard this story before, you may miss the significance of the phrase *He ran down the road to meet him*. Jesus is introducing us to God. He is saying that this is how God is. He is like the father who, without judgment or consideration, runs down the road to greet the very son who had insulted him.

There was a day I finally realized the point Jesus was making, and my heart was filled with relief and joy. This is how God is. That was incredible for me because I was like the son. I had no question about that. What a wonderful introduction to the love and forgiving generosity of God.

The son tried to apologize but the father did not need an apology. He could have been angry, rejecting or cynical about the return. Most fathers would look down the road, see the son in the distance and think, "Here he comes for another loan." Not this father. He opened his arms and heart and said, "Here is my son. He was dead, now he is alive. Let's celebrate."

It should not be difficult for anyone who binges on food to identify with this errant son. How many times have you watched your food intake carefully for days, only to suddenly lose control and gorge yourself on anything available?

It is as if you lose time and space and wake up just like this young man in the pig-pen of your destructive behavior, angry, hurt and in physical pain. You hate yourself for the indulgence, yet you have no way to release yourself from the guilt. Your emotional reaction will often produce a repeat of the same self-destructive behavior and a return visit to the hell of food addiction.

The way out is to identify with the son and then allow yourself to be introduced to this incredible father. His love, generosity and willingness to embrace you and welcome you home will make the difference. This introduction will help break the painful and destructive cycle of binge, self-hate, then binge again.

But Jesus is not the only source of proper introduction to God. Here is a story I have borrowed from the

Zen Buddhists. It is similar to the story of the good father.

I first encountered Zen in my twenties. A friend gave me a book of Zen teachings and stories entitled *Zen Bones, Zen Flesh,* edited by Paul Reps. I have read regularly from its worn pages ever since. Zen's straight-to-the-point clarity brings a sophisticated simplicity to many issues that would otherwise remain confused and clouded in mystery. This book contains one of my favorite tales.

One point of clarification: Zen does not profess a belief in God in the Western sense. In fact, many Zen practitioners would say it is more a philosophy or a point of view than a religion. Its goal is not salvation but enlightenment.

Many students of Zen may be surprised that I use the following story to illustrate the nature of God. But it is my opinion that a Zen master would agree this simple, but powerful, tale does introduce us to the true nature of the universe. In Western language, we could easily translate "universe" as "God." See what you think. Here is my version of the master at the wall (my title).

Centuries ago in Japan there was a zendo (Zen school) that was led by an enlightened master. Like the masters of all zendos, he had the power of life and death over his students. The study of Zen was considered to be a matter that required total commitment, and each student accepted the master's complete authority.

At this school there was a student who was a rebel. Though he loved and respected his teacher, he had an uncontrollable desire for fun. Many nights after curfew, he would sneak out of bed, climb the garden wall and spend the night carousing in the nearby village. He imagined that his teacher was unaware of his infidelity, and he continued his antics for weeks.

Finally, the master, who had known all along, decided it was time to put an end to the rebellion and teach his student a lesson. He waited until the young man had gone for the night, then placed himself strategically under the wall where the student had always left a stool to step on.

The story does not say how long the master waited. But any Zen master would have no trouble meditating quietly for hours. Finally, the half-drunk young man returned. He climbed over the wall and, without looking, placed his foot where the stool had always been. This time, however, he stepped on his teacher's head. When he realized what he had done, he fell to the ground in horror and humiliation. Trembling with fear, he waited to be killed or at least ejected from the school. The master's response changed his life forever.

Quietly, without anger or judgment, the master said, "You must be careful. You will catch cold on a night like this." Then he turned and walked away. From that day forth, the young man became the most devoted student in the zendo.

Spiritual truth is apparently universal. This story has the same essential message that is contained in Jesus' parable about the good father. The Zen master responded to the student with such unprecedented insight and compassion that he transformed his heart. This is the mark of a true spiritual master.

A normal teacher's reaction would have been judgment and condemnation. The student had clearly broken the rules. His nightly trips were indefensible, and placing his foot upon his teacher's head was unforgivable. *But judgment and condemnation never transformed anyone's life.* Every true and enlightened spiritual master knows that.

It is the mark of a master to be able to respond to the difficulties present in human nature with the healing and compassionate nature of divinity. It always produces a miracle. It is always a proper introduction to God.

One more story from my favorite spiritual mentor, Rumi. This one may be read in its entirety in *The One-Handed Basket Weaver,* edited by Coleman Barks. Here is my condensed version.

Once there was a Sufi saint who lived near an orchard. As a symbol of his total surrender to God, he vowed to eat only fruit the wind blew off the full branches. For many months, the wind was strong and he ate his fill. He thanked God daily for his nurture and care.

Then, without warning, the wind stopped. For days, not a leaf stirred and not a single fruit dropped to the ground. The saint became concerned. His vow prevented him from plucking fruit, and he was beginning to starve. He struggled and suffered and prayed incessantly, to no avail. Finally, in desperation, he broke his vow and picked a fruit. It was delicious.

At the moment the saint was eating the forbidden fruit, a group of thieves was robbing the orchard. A squad of soldiers arrived and arrested them and took the saint as well, confusing him with the outlaws. They administered swift justice and began to chop off a hand and foot from each transgressor.

They cut a hand from the saint's body before they realized their terrible mistake. When they threw themselves on the ground in grief, the saint immediately forgave them. He indicated that he had broken his vow and losing his hand was a just result. Then he left the orchard.

Arriving in another village, the saint took up a new profession to support himself. He became a basket weaver. He selected a secluded hut so no one could see the miracle that occurred every time he worked. But someone finally peeked through his window and told the village what was happening.

Every time the one-handed saint sat down to weave a basket, a mysterious spirit hand would appear to help him. He was now full partners with and completely surrendered to God. As Rumi would say, he had been blessed by the loss of his hand. God himself had engineered the apparent tragedy in order to become intimately bound to his servant.

I have chosen three stories about indulgence to facilitate this introduction. I could tell a thousand more. My point is this: Effective prayer occurs when we pray to a God we love and trust. If you do not completely love God, you must not blame yourself. You simply need a better introduction.

Let's return to the original question: "Is God really interested in my weight loss?" I hope my stories have convinced you that God cares about every aspect of your existence. His love is complete and detailed. He is fully aware of your needs. He sees you from afar when you begin the journey home. He watches over you when you go "over the wall" and knows the intimate and silent cries of your heart.

Yes, God cares about your weight loss. Absolutely, completely, no question about it.

### Do I Have to Believe in God to Pray?

Americans are "poll addicted." We take a poll for everything. Recently, I saw one that indicated over 90 percent of Americans believe in God. That poll may be accurate, but it does not mean that we also believe in prayer. We think God exists, but many of us are not sure he wants to hear what we want or need.

I am convinced of this because of my own "anecdotal polls"—administered unscientifically from my own experience. Hundreds of clients, workshop participants and e-mailers have asked me the same question: *"Do I have to believe in God to pray?"*

My answer reflects one more amazing aspect of the real nature of God. *No. You do not have to believe in God to pray. Furthermore, you do not have to believe in God to get an answer to your prayer.*

To explain myself, I have to become a Sufi for a moment and use a phrase I like to call a mantra. This is a

Hindu term, but it seems to accurately describe the Sufi's use of the words *"La'illaha il' Allahu,"* which means, *"There is no reality but God. There is only God."* To the Sufis, and to me, this is a fact. God is all, and all is God. Nothing exists outside of God. In a sense, we might say God is like the ocean and we are like fish. The ocean is all around and through us. It is in every cell of our bodies and in every direction we turn. We are natural creatures of the sea, and we cannot swim beyond its boundaries.

Does it matter, then, if a fish does not believe in the ocean? Does the existence of the ocean or its care and nurture of the fish depend on belief? Absolutely not. Neither does the existence or care of God depend on our acceptance or denial of His existence.

It also follows that a Conscious Ocean (God) would be continually aware of every fish that swims in its embrace. How then could it not hear the fish's cries for help? I believe this is also true for every one of us. God hears our prayers whether we are sure of His existence or not.

What kind of God would ignore a creature that He is so intimately bound to? Rumi says He is closer to us than our own heartbeat. How much closer can He get? Does He hear and respond? Of course. We can count on it.

Every time I am asked the question about belief and prayer, I have the same response. You don't need belief to pray. Just pray. Ask honestly for what you need. Pray like this: *"God, if you are there and you care about me, then please answer my prayer."* Then, open your heart and mind to receive the answer. Nothing creates belief like answered prayer.

### Praying for Weight Loss

Another recent poll reported that over 55 percent of Americans are overweight. One has only to sit on a bench at a local mall to confirm this fact. We like to eat and have to eat, and many of us are addicted to eating. Therefore, we are fat.

In addition to being dedicated to excessive food consumption, we are just as addicted to dieting. Sadly, most of us cannot keep the weight off. We suffer to lose a few pounds and then quickly regain it, often with the additional baggage of self-hate.

We hate ourselves for being fat and for not having the self-discipline we think is required to be a successful dieter. The cycle is viciously destructive and leads us deeper into a blurry and seemingly hopeless mess of obesity. It would appear that only a miracle could solve this problem. I believe that prayer will move us toward that miracle.

The second most-asked question I hear about prayer and weight loss is this: *"Is it O.K. to ask God to help me lose weight?"* The question is simple but implies important information about the questioner's theology and self-concept. Both need to be addressed before a prayer can be prayed.

As I mentioned above, self-hate and low self-esteem

almost always accompany obesity. (Which, for the purposes of this book, I define as being chronically twenty-five or more pounds overweight.) We hate being fat, and we hate ourselves for staying that way. It is an American value and illness that we are spreading around the planet, and it is one of the many curses that emerge from the dark side of affluence.

Self-hate blocks our ability to act positively on our own behalf. How, then, could we institute and maintain healthy eating patterns if we hate who we are? More importantly, how could we expect God to care about us if we hate ourselves? The problem is that many of us confuse our self-concept with God's concept. *We actually assume God is incapable of loving us because we don't love ourselves.*

This tragic assumption often stands between us and healing. It manifests as a self-limiting and ultimately self-destructive form of logic.

"I don't love myself, therefore God cannot love me."

"If God cannot love me, then I cannot ask him for help."

This kind of logic is the central reason most people do not pray for weight loss. In fact, it is the central reason many of us do not pray at all. We restrict our prayers not from lack of belief in God but from lack of a sense of deserving. We think we are not worthy.

In order to pray earnestly and consistently for weight loss, we need to find a bridge that will carry us over the "chasm of unworthiness." It is deep and extremely broad, and we usually need every bit of help we can get.

Psychology provides us with numerous processes and techniques that can make a great difference on our journey to worthiness. I have explored many of these personally and professionally over the last thirty years. I have discovered that something more is required to span the incredibly expansive chasm of unworthiness, and that is spirituality. We need God to take us the final step.

I want to be very clear so that I am not misunderstood. *Psychology is extremely important and necessary for inner healing, and inner healing is necessary for sustained weight loss.* Many spiritually-oriented weight-loss programs lose sight of this fact and persuade their followers that "God is all you need." They seem to fear the sometimes messy, painful and dark revelations that psychology exposes. Then they blame their constituents for insufficient faith when weight is not lost or returns.

I am not demeaning the role of psychology in the process of inner healing and sustained weight loss. I am saying, however, that it cannot take us across the chasm of unworthiness all by itself. I know this truth not from theory but from personal experience.

I have tried everything psychology had to offer, and it has been good, healing and extremely helpful. But somewhere near the middle of the chasm, its bridge stopped. It could take me no further. I needed another helper and, to tell you the truth, I hated it.

I didn't hate God, mind you. I hated what God told me I had to do next: Surrender.

For me, and I imagine for many other seekers of healing and growth, psychology gave me a sense of control. I could walk under my own power into the dark side of my psyche with the sword and shield of psychological theory and technique and face the demons and dragons that resided there. I could read and journal and do internal dialogues and analyze my dreams, talk to my therapists (they have been legion), scream, rage, sob and laugh on uncountable workshops and numerous groups and even stand naked before fellow seekers and talk about what I hated and loved about my body. I could do all of these things and all of these things made a difference but they could not finish the bridge.

Then God sent me another dream. I say God sent the dream because I firmly believe all dreams originate in that divine presence that is at the deepest center of who we are. The Hindus call it atman, or the divine self. They knew it long before the birth of the other great religions. The rest of us have created our own words for it, but for me the word that describes it best is God.

God creates and sends dreams, and they are all ultimately meant for helping and healing. But that is another book. Here is the dream that guided me across the chasm.

*I am alone in the middle of a vast ocean. I am clinging desperately to a piece of broken wood. It is part of the shattered remains of a boat I was sailing on. The boat has exploded and left me afloat and stranded with no help in sight.*

*I look around and become intensely aware that rescue is not going to occur. This is it. I am alone and on my own with only a broken board to hold on to. In that moment I decide I will let go and sink into the ocean. Giving up will be better than floating hopelessly in the middle of a desert of water.*

*I let go and immediately begin to descend into the quickly darkening water. I sink deeper and deeper. I am aware that the light grows dimmer and dimmer until it totally disappears. I continue to sink deeper and deeper into the darkness. I wait to run out of air and die.*

*Then, without warning, I come to the ocean floor. It is white sand, and I can see. As soon as my feet touch bottom, a man comes out of a nearby cave and does something to me, and I can breathe. He disappears.*

*I turn and see the sand has become a white path leading off into the distance. In that moment I am clear that I am supposed to walk that path. As I begin to walk, I wake up.*

To me, the dream was obviously about surrender. It was telling me, with elegant images, that it was time to let go and allow myself to sink into that which is deep, vast and initially dark. I could trust that something would be there to guide me, but I would have no control after I made the decision to let go. The theme of surrender was upon me once again. I had no choice.

What does all this have to do with weight loss, self-hate and the feeling of unworthiness? Everything. It prepared me for a transforming encounter with something I had considered irrelevant since I finished seminary: the First Commandment.

## The First Commandment: Antidote to Self-Hate

From the moment I became a teenager, I ceased to be a fan of the Ten Commandments. They seemed to be rigid rules created and enforced by an angry and judgmental God. I was always afraid of that God and had many of the same feelings about quite a few of his followers. They appeared to rejoice every time I made a mistake, and love and compassion were not high on their list of values. When they showed up, I usually went the other way, so I felt little connection with them or their commandments.

I felt that the First Commandment . . . "Thou shalt have no other gods before me" . . . was particularly irrelevant to contemporary life, because the gods, idols and graven images that plagued the Israelites were nonexistent in Western society. Nobody was building golden images of baal in local parking lots, so I figured I was safe.

I am aware that many of my religious colleagues would argue that Baal has changed form and now appears disguised as materialism, success, drugs, fame, and so on. For me, these were not gods or signs of evil but important issues to address as part of my growth and inner healing.

I knew they were there, and I faced them as best I could, but they did not seem to have divine power over my life. They were not gods that came between me and the true God. I had yet to meet that illusive character, and I never expected him to appear inside my own heart and mind.

It was only after many years of hard and very productive inner work that I finally came to the end of the bridge that psychology had so effectively built. I stood at the precipice and regretfully realized I could no longer control the process. Something new and fundamentally different had to occur, and it would not come from me.

It was here that I began to become aware that my path was blocked by a powerful force, a force more dynamic and dominating than anything I had ever encountered: my ego.

The term "ego" has become the property of popular culture and has many uses and interpretations, some superficial and some deeply meaningful. I am using it here to mean the following.

The ego represents the clearest and most encompassing definition of who I think I am. It tells me who Matthew is, what he has been and who he is capable of being. It is a necessary function. Without an intact ego, I cannot relate effectively to my world. Its existence is a result of normal, natural developmental processes. The ego is not bad, dangerous or evil. It is, in fact, necessary to healthy psychological and spiritual growth, *until one comes to the end of the bridge.*

Once we come to the end of that bridge, we need to change our relationship to the ego or we will remain stranded in the middle of the chasm. It is here that we must learn to do the opposite of everything that has gotten us this far. We must let go of the ego and surrender to

God's definition of who we are. We must come to worship a new God.

As to the issue of worthiness, egos can become false and dangerous gods. It is the ego that takes a look at our history and list of failures and says, *"Listen to me. I know you better than anyone. I know all your dark secrets and nasty habits. You can't fool me. All these people who say they are your friends and counselors don't know what I know. You wish you could trust them and believe you are worthy of love, forgiveness, healing and all the other good things they promise. But I know better. You are not worth it, and you never will be."*

This inner voice comes to us with the power of a god and effectively shuts the door on love and healing. It blocks our ability to receive the transforming embrace of the father who runs down the road to greet us, the master who refuses to condemn us for stepping on his head and the loving God who hears the true message of prayer in our hearts.

This god, this ego, that defines the limits of our worthiness, is the one that tells us that weight loss is an absurd topic for prayer. It also says we don't deserve to lose weight or that we are idiots for imagining we are worthy of the attention of He Who Creates the Universe. Too often, we bow before this force without realizing it has become not the carrier of reasonable self-definition or of eternal truth, but a false god that is not capable of carrying us one step further on our journey.

When I came to this realization, I was ready to see an entirely new and relevant understanding of the First Commandment. It was time to take back the authority I had given to my ego and hand it to the only Power that could carry me across the abyss of unworthiness.

My ego's definition of my value and essential nature was too limited and constricted to allow me to receive the transforming love that wanted to embrace me. It was time to surrender and allow my ego to drown in the dark waters of abandon.

I, my ego, could not be allowed to control or limit the goodness that wanted to engulf me. That god had to die. It could only be killed by an attitude and behavior that was totally contrary to its direction and nature: Losing control of my self-definition and surrendering that definition to God. It was time to allow the true and compassionate God to tell me who I am and what I am worth.

Herein lies the secret to truly effective and transforming prayer. God always hears and responds to our prayers, but self-imposed limits dictated by our egos prevent us from receiving the answers. The First Commandment is the antidote to this dilemma.

Remembering and honoring the First Commandment will bring us to a new attitude about the ego. It will allow us to begin the difficult process of releasing ourselves from the domination of ego definition and surrendering to God's life—changing our vision of our true worth.

There is no miracle more astounding than this. We are not the person we were sure we were. We had no idea of the extent of our beauty or value. To paraphrase the good father in the parable, *"We were dead. Now we are alive."*

Finally, let's remember the question once again: *"Is it*

O.K. to ask God to help me to lose weight?" Your answer is, an obvious and hopeful "Yes."

> What if your ego was the only thing between you and the greatest happiness you could ever imagine? Would you ask God to bypass it for just one moment?

## Seven

# SPIRITUAL DEPRIVATION AND THE GOD INSTINCT

"Sit down in this circle.

Quit acting like a wolf, and feel
the Shepherd's Love filling you.

At night your Beloved wanders.
Don't take pain-killers.

Tonight, no consolations.
And don't eat.

Close your mouth against food.
Taste the Lover's mouth in yours."

—Jelaludin Rumi

In the mid-1980s, my wife and I took a nine-month sabbatical and moved to the San Francisco area. We spent the majority of our time pursuing both traditional and non-traditional spiritual practices. In the process, we met many interesting individuals who were deeply committed in their search for God. One of those opened my mind to a concept that is central for long-term weight loss.

My new friend and I were sitting in a small coffee shop in Palo Alto, a lovely and affluent community that is the home of Stanford University. I was drinking coffee and he was sipping herbal tea. Near the end of our conversation he told me he had recently returned from a six-month stay at an ashram (religious community) in India.

I naively asked "*what it was like to spend half a year in a place so deprived and then arrive here in the lap of prosperity.*" His response opened me to an obvious reality.

"*I have been struck not by the material affluence of Americans but by their spiritual poverty. In India, spirituality is a part of everyday life. They are as committed to and involved with their spiritual pursuits as Americans are to their material ones. Americans are as spiritually deprived as Indians are materially deprived. Since I have returned from India, I am painfully aware of this and am amazed I never saw it before. As a society, we are suffering tremendously from this deprivation and we don't even notice it.*"

We discussed this concept at length for about an hour. I have not seen him since and I do not remember his name. Sometimes I think of him as an angel, who ap-

pears long enough to deliver a package that makes a difference in life, then disappears. Wherever he went, I wish
him well. He left me with a new awareness that has positively influenced my personal and professional lives.

Since that encounter, I have been increasingly aware
of the reality of spiritual deprivation. I have also come to
believe it is a major contributor to the "American plague"
of obesity. We are overweight because we are starving for
something we confuse with food. An essential and instinctive part of us is deprived and demands attention
and we try to satiate it with pizza, pop, chocolate and
chips. Sadly, our food indulgences only increase the spiritual deficit *and* our waistlines.

### The God Instinct

> "*Where we locate Spirit: This is the great question of our times,
> is it not . . . the one location of Spirit that damages none, em-
> braces all, and announces itself with the simplest of clarity,
> which leaves no places left untouched by care nor cuts its em-
> brace for a chosen few; neither does it hide its face in the shad-
> ows of true believers, nor take up residence on a chosen piece of
> real estate, but rather looks out from the very person now read-
> ing these lines, too obvious to ignore, too simple to describe, too
> easy to believe.*
> *In the eye of the Spirit we will all meet, and I will find you
> there, and you me, and the miracle is that we will find each
> other at all. And the fact that we do is one of the simplest
> proofs, no doubt, of God's insistent existence.*"

—Ken Wilber

It should be obvious that humans have a deeply ingrained need for a relationship with the Divine. Archeologists consistently find religious artifacts at the center of life of all ancient peoples. But science has been wary of theology for centuries and has hesitated to expound on this historical reality.

Given the often irrational and violent reactions of the organized church to perceived heresy, I cannot fault science for its hesitancy. However, it remains a fact that human beings have something more than a predilection toward religion. We are instinctively religious.

Dr. C. A. Meier, a physician, psychiatrist and Jungian analyst has written a book entitled *SOUL AND BODY: Essays on the Theories of C.G. Jung*. In his insightful and provocative chapter, "Psychology and Religion," he explores Jung's groundbreaking discoveries about man's natural religiosity.

> *"Jung in his work discovered what he calls a religious factor in nature. He found it in dreams, and dreams are products of nature. On this basis it appears that there is such a thing as a religious instinct . . . Since 1912, when he published SYMBOLS OF TRANSFORMATION, and more particularly since 1937, when he gave the Terry lectures, he has provided evidence for the fact that the religious factor is something* sui generis*—that it exists in the same way other instincts exist, which means they cannot be reduced to anything more elementary."*

Dr. Meier goes on to make a second and equally profound statement often quoted in the Jungian community of analysts.

> *"Jung said he never really cured a patient in the second half of life unless, in the course of treatment, that person found access to the religious function. As this statement was made as a result of Jung's vast experience, we simply are compelled to believe it."*

Simply translated, Dr. Meier is saying Carl Jung, one of the greatest minds of the last century, was convinced about two realities.

1. Being religious is essential, basic and instinctive to human nature.
2. Mental and emotional problems cannot be cured (in the second half of life) without meaningful attention to the religious function.

In everyday religious language this means humans are created in the image of God. We are specifically constructed, physically, mentally and emotionally, to have a relationship with That Which Is Divine. It also means our mental and emotional difficulties, which are directly related to weight problems, cannot be cured without attention to this essential need.

This "God instinct" is elementary to what makes us function as natural human beings. Dr. Meier uses the

Latin phrase—*sui generis*—to describe our God instinct as irreducible, meaning it is what it is and is not representative of something deeper or more basic to the organism. *The God instinct is as basic and necessary to human existence as the survival instinct.*

It is no wonder Jung also discovered psychological cures were not possible after an individual passed through the spiritually activating passage of mid-life without attention to a meaningful relationship with Divine Presence. I would go one step further and say many mid-life difficulties, including weight gain, are the result of long-term neglect of the needs related to the God instinct.

We do not have to rely only on the word of doctors Meier and Jung as to the existence of the God instinct. All the great religious traditions throughout human history reflect this reality. The existence of the traditions themselves is testimony to something essential to human need. We must be religious. Forms, of course, are as varied as humans, but the deep-seated drive to connect with a Divine Source is constant and dominant. It requires attention and if neglected will create its own powerful and unavoidable symptoms.

Finally I am not saying that all mental, emotional and physical (weight-related) problems are a result of spiritual deprivation. Ilness of many kinds and obesity appear in the lives of spiritually developed persons and are not a result of lack of attention to their God instinct. I am saying, from personal experience, however, that consistent neglect of this basic and central human need is dangerous. It will cause a variety of unpleasant symptoms that can and do include chronic weight problems.

> *What if prayer was as natural as breathing? What if it required no thought or preparation? What if your life and the way you live it is your most powerful prayer? How will it be answered?*

## Spiritual Deprivation

Once we accept the reality of the God instinct, we are prepared to seriously consider the results that occur when we neglect its messages and needs. My angelic friend was correct. As a whole, our American society is spiritually deprived. We are awash in religiosity, religious belief and religious organization but we lack true spiritual experience and nurture. As the poet said, "water, water, everywhere but not a drop to drink."

Simply being religious does not nurture the soul and an unnurtured soul can generate powerful energies that often imitate hunger. I will explore this weight-producing reality in a moment, but first I want to make this point.

More than 90% of Americans profess a belief in God and most are affiliated with organized religion. Sadly, this plus a dollar won't even get them a cup of Starbucks coffee. One of my mentors, Werner Erhard, used to say, "understanding was the booby prize." I would like to offer my update of his insightful comment in the context of this conversation, "Belief is the booby prize."

Belief without experience is like paper without a pen or a body without a pulse. America has yet to fully wake up to this truth and suffers greatly from its religious naivete. One of the most spiritually deprived hours of the week is 11 o'clock Sunday morning. Immersed in frozen ritual, safe sermonizing, hollow and untested beliefs, social event announcements, irrelevant moralizing and thinly-disguised contemporary advertising and entertainment techniques, the average congregant has no opportunity for an experience of Divine Presence.

In his book "The Adventure of Self-Discovery" Stanislav Grof quotes his friend, and professor of religion, Walter Houston Clark, as follows:

> *"He (Clark) said that much of mainstream religion reminded him of a vaccination. One goes to church and gets 'a little something that then protects him or her against the real thing.' Thus, many people believe that regular attendance of church on Sundays and holidays, saying the prayers, and listening to the sermons is sufficient for being truly religious. This false sense of having already arrived then prevents them from starting on a journey of spiritual discovery."*

Millions of sincere seekers trust their starving hearts and souls to the care of established American religion. Every week, they are promised redemption, salvation, spiritual guidance and an introduction to God that will fill their impoverished hearts. At the end of the day, they are left with little more than an uncontrollable urge to eat everything in sight.

Lest you decide I am biased, I would like to speak briefly about the community of seekers we call New Age. Since the early 1970s, I have been an enthusiastic student of many New Age doctrines, methodologies, organizations and teachers. During that time I lived in Boston, New York, Los Angeles, San Francisco, Hawaii and Florida. There is little that is central or peripheral to this movement I have not experienced. I received value from much of it and am not demeaning its essence. I simply want to focus, for a moment, on its limitations.

The New Age movement is composed in large part of individuals who felt betrayed, damaged and disillusioned with organized American religion. They left church and synagogue in search of a personal and life-nurturing experience of God. They are no more "flakey" or neurotic than the traditional religious establishment. They found the courage to seek Spirit outside the safe boundaries of dogma and habit. Many of them, to some degree, feel they have found meaningful answers to their heartfelt questions and would never consider returning to the spiritual emptiness of their past.

Ironically, many New Agers have more faith in the statement "Seek and you shall find" than the average churchgoer. They have allowed their hearts to lead in search of truth and this sincerity has often paid off. But even with these payoffs, there remains a price that is relevant to our discussion about spiritual deprivation.

As a whole, the New Age movement lacks depth and discipline of mind and heart. It has little appreciation for what theologian Matthew Fox calls the "via negativa." It cannot provide guidance into the dark areas of life. Reacting to the neurotic judgment and negativity so constantly taught and practiced by traditional religion, New Agers resist even the slightest journey into their inner darkness.

The New Age has a polarized obsession with "Light" and positive energy. This leaves it with little more than the straw swords of affirmations, crystals and six-packs of audio tapes that promise total transformation in three days to fight the monsters of grief, self-hate and deep spiritual emptiness.

In addition to its typical avoidance of inner pain and darkness, the New Age movement often fosters spiritual dilettantism. This tendency has generated many individuals who are jacks of all spiritual paths but masters of none. When pushed and shoved by the rigors of true spiritual growth, they opt not for commitment and self-sacrifice but for another, "less stressful," modality. Ultimately, they find themselves as impoverished and starving for God as their traditionally religious neighbors.

Am I saying Americans are severely spiritually deprived? Yes I am. Am I saying this deprivation cuts across traditional and New Age lines? Absolutely. Am I saying spiritual deprivation contributes to numerous diseases and unpleasant symptoms, including overeating and obesity? No question about it.

*Eight*

# SPIRITUAL DEPRIVATION AND HUNGER

*"When one loss causes a greedy panic,
then more losses are liable to come."*

—Jelaludin Rumi

If we accept that our need for divine contact is instinctive, then we must also accept the neglect of that instinct will have significant consequences. Traditional religion has most frequently acknowledged this reality but has located the "payment" (hell) in the afterlife. I do not consider obesity to be a punishment from God, but I am convinced that overeating is often a result of spiritual deprivation.

Individuals who report being spiritually deprived often say they "feel empty" in the lower abdomen or stomach. To a New Ager or Hindu, this would be designated as the second or third chakra. This experience can be mentally, emotionally and physically intense, even painful. In many cases I have observed, including my own, these symptoms can be easily confused with hunger. In extreme cases, they appear as starvation and will provoke the same panic.

*Those who became spiritually deprived are literally experiencing a hunger for God.* To the average American, the solution is material food, and for a while it works. The painful sensation of God-hunger dissipates but soon returns and activates the self-defeating eating pattern. We become physically fat instead of being filled with the spirit.

In her small but insightful book, *Addiction to Perfection,* Marion Woodman makes the following observations.

*"Jung believed that religion is one of man's instincts, a natural need that must, therefore, be satisfied. In our world, where the institutionalized sacred is being increasingly profaned, compensation takes over . . . (but) the muffin cannot*

*replace the divine wafer, nor can alcohol replace the divine spirit, nor can starving replace a religious fast. When our animal and spiritual signs are confused, bizarre behavior results. The emptiness gnaws and the wolf prowls until some kind of ritual is performed. If it is a compulsive ritual, it can become nothing less than a hurricane swirling its victim headlong into unconsciousness. The natural spiritual hunger, if it is not fed by the sacred, is trapped in the demonic."*

Tragically, many of us are caught in the dangerous process that Dr. Woodman describes. Our "natural spiritual hunger" arises, and we naively attempt to satisfy it with muffins. But muffins are no substitute for meaningful spiritual nurturing, and we are plunged into an even deeper deprivation that erupts as compulsive, addictive behavior (food binges, for example).

When Dr. Woodman uses the word "demonic" she is not referring to entities like the main character in the movie, *The Exorcist*. She is describing an energy that is much more pervasive and potentially destructive. It emerges in each of us when we neglect the desperate calls of our spiritual instinct. If we allow ourselves to become spiritually starved, a ravenous wolf appears and drives us to bizarre behavior.

Jesus fasted for forty days before he began his ministry. He was obviously aware material and spiritual food could be confused. It is no accident that in the midst of his fast he uttered the well-known phrase *"Man does not live by bread alone but by every word that comes out of the mouth of God."*

This statement is an eloquent reminder that human survival has more than one source. Bread is necessary and is acknowledged, but "bread alone" cannot sustain our existence. We must also have spiritual nurture, connection and guidance. The great Christian mystic, Meister Eckhart, speaks to this issue in this fashion: *"Our bodily food is changed into us, but our spiritual food changes us into itself."*

The food of the spirit, according to Eckhart, does something that material food cannot. It performs a unique and necessary function that nurtures and transforms our minds and hearts. It gives us food for the long journey of the soul.

It is no accident that fasting and careful food management are central to the guidelines and practices of most religious communities. Experienced spiritual seekers are aware of the potential confusion between spiritual deprivation and hunger. We would be wise to heed their warnings and pay more attention to our own symptoms. We must learn to tell the difference.

I have discovered the easiest way to make this crucial distinction is by asking a simple question on a daily basis until the answer is clear.

*"Am I spiritually deprived?"*

If a clear answer does not appear immediately, you may want to use the checklist I have provided below.

## A Spiritual Deprivation Checklist

I am firmly convinced that most Americans are spiritually deprived. Chances are you are like the rest of us. So don't use this list to condemn yourself. Use it to motivate a new search for a connection to God. If you think of items that are not listed, add them and attend to them.

If you answer "yes" to all the questions on this list, you are doing extremely well in the spiritual nurturing department. If you answer "no" to one or more, you will have a good idea of the areas of your spiritual life that need attention.

1. *I spend time daily or weekly in nature, and when I do I often feel connected to an energy or source greater than myself.*

2. *I often remember my dreams and regularly experience them as a source of divine guidance.*

3. *I read spiritually-oriented literature on a daily or weekly basis.*

4. *I practice one or more religious rituals daily or weekly.*

5. *I have contact daily or weekly with a community of like-minded believers.*

6. *I regularly take time to be alone, without distraction, and listen to my deeper self.*

7. *I meditate in one form or another on a daily or weekly basis.*

8. *I see the daily appearance of divine guidance in my normal life routines and relationships.*

9. *I have a clear sense that my life has purpose and meaning that is in concert with divine will.*
10. *I constantly learn important spiritual lessons from both the positive and negative events that occur in my daily life.*
11. *I pray daily.*
12. *I feel known and deeply loved by the Divine Lover.*

If your answer is "Yes, I am spiritually deprived," what must you do to find spiritual nurturing both immediately and regularly? Blind trust in traditional and New Age religious organizations will not guarantee an authentic encounter with God. So what can you do that will work?

*You can pray.*

### Prayer as Soul Food

Prayer is a natural human function. Every human being, child or adult, can do it. We all know how to pray, just as we know how to breathe. We carry this ability with us wherever we go and whoever we are.

Prayer gives us access to God, immediately and without pomp or circumstance. We do not need ritual, dogma, priest, guru or sacred book. God is closer to us than our own breath. We only need to ask Him for help.

Once we ask for divine guidance, we must look for and expect direction. God is always faithful and will always lead us to the people, places and things that will ensure and expand spiritual growth and nurture. I have seen this uncomplicated process work so consistently in

my life and the lives of others that I unhesitatingly recommend it to everyone.

Recently, I spent a year as the spiritual director of a
local treatment center for chemically dependent adults.
My job was to conduct a weekly, two-hour "spirituality
group" for twenty-five to thirty young, highly intelligent,
world-weary addicts. They had no tolerance for stock or
simplistic answers to their sincere questions about God.
Most of them felt burned and abandoned by the religious
establishment and were in desperate need of honest and
practical information about how to find God.

I came to treasure my time with these amazing people. For most of them, addiction had brought them to the
edge of survival. Scarred wrists and tales of overdoses
abounded. Life itself was in constant question. *"Why
should I stay in this life? Who will help me? Why has God let
this happen to me?"*

As painful as their lives were, their addiction had
brought them to questions many of us never seriously ask.
The answers, if relevant and meaningful, could change
their lives forever. There was no margin for error.

A life crisis always tests the depth of one's spiritual
development. There is a story that circulates in twelve-
step circles that best illustrates this truth.

A minister was once invited to an AA meeting to discuss the difference between religion and spirituality. He
droned on dryly about the subject for half an hour until
an old and grizzled alcoholic stood up in the back of the
room and interrupted his lecture. *"Reverend, I would like to
give you my definition of the difference between religion and*

*spirituality. Religion, sir, is for all you people who are afraid of going to hell. Spirituality is for those of us who have already been there."*

Every patient in every treatment center in America understands this story. Talk is cheap for someone in extreme pain. A real experience of the loving care and guidance of God is what makes the difference. Tell us something that works, or shut up and sit down.

I am not a chemically dependent person, unless we include food. I am, however, a veteran of many battles with extreme stress. I am intimately acquainted with hopelessness, rage, fear, disappointment, loss, humiliation and other painful emotions. I would have been happy to avoid all of these dark teachers, but they have left me with an invaluable legacy. I know prayer works.

When spiritually desperate addicts asked how to find God, I always gave them my best and truest answer. *"If you want to find God in a way that will be real and meaningful and trustable, then you must pray. Just pray and do your best to open yourself to receive the answers that will come."*

You may or may not be an addict. You may or may not be in the midst of a life crisis. But you are probably struggling with the pain and frustration of weight gain and all that has come to mean to you. I will give you the same advice I have given thousands of others.

The antidote to spiritual deprivation is prayer. Pray for help and guidance and nurture and love and anything else you need. Then open your mind and heart to receive the specific and graceful answers that will appear.

If you need to lose weight, pray for weight loss. Your

prayers will lead you to everything you need and more. Your deprived spirit will flourish and your hunger will subside as the nourishment arrives. Nothing is more satisfying than answered prayer.

> *What if your belly hunger is really spiritual hunger? What if your food panic is really spiritual panic? How will this realization affect your prayer?*

# Nine

# PRAYER AND FOOD ADDICTION

*"This is how a human being can change:*

*There's a worm addicted to eating*
*grape leaves.*

*Suddenly he wakes up.*
*Call it Grace——whatever——something*
*wakes him, and he's no longer*
*a worm.*

*He's the entire vineyard,*
*and the orchard, too, the fruit, the trunks,*
*a growing wisdom and joy*
*that doesn't need*
*to devour."*

—Jelaludin Rumi

Are you a food addict? If you believed you were a food addict, would it change you in any way? How do you decide if you are an addict? What are the criteria?

I have attached a food addiction checklist below, but there is a simple question that can produce an accurate answer: *Have you been at least twenty-five pounds overweight for a year or more?* If your answer is yes, you probably have a food addiction.

Food addiction affects more Americans than any other addiction. It is far more pervasive than alcoholism, drug addiction or addictions related to smoking, gambling, sex or even shopping. At least half of all Americans are food addicts. But almost no one admits to it. We ignore the symptoms and actually celebrate the addiction.

We love to fill our commercials with throngs of smiling and joyous people engaging in food orgies. We include excessive amounts of food in every aspect of our lives. We eat while driving, working, riding in airplanes, exercising, having sex and even sitting on the toilet. We think we cannot function without food and are insulted if someone forgets to provide it. Are we food addicts? Yes, but few are ready to admit it.

Admitting food addiction is the first step toward recovery. We cannot attend to something we will not acknowledge. Once we have faced the reality, we can begin to use the resources that will support our healing. You already know if you are addicted to food. But in case you need a little more clarity, I have included my Food Addiction Checklist. Take a few moments to read the list.

I think you will have an answer before you get to the last question.

### The Food Addiction Checklist

I have created this checklist from my experience with my own food addiction, and from many thousands of workshop participants, individuals who have responded to my columns and individual counseling clients. I am sure there are signs and symptoms I have not included. The 12 questions go directly to the point. If you answer yes to even three of the 12, you are probably food addicted.

If the answers reveal an addiction, remember this truth: Having a food addiction does not make you a bad or worthless human being. You are a worthwhile, valuable person who has a problem with food . . . and you have plenty of company. Lots of us are food addicted.

Remember, self-hate is not the goal here. Telling the truth about your addiction will be a giant step toward meaningful recovery. The task before you is to face the facts and get on with the process of healing.

## ARE YOU A FOOD ADDICT?

1. *I have been at least twenty-five pounds overweight for a year or more.* (I have not included height or gender factors here because you know whether you have been overweight. You also know if it is a chronic problem.)

2. *Eating is most often the "high point" of my day.* (Do you start thinking about food well before meals? Do you get excited by the idea of a special meal? Do you feel this way often? Is there anything in your life that gives you more pleasure than food?)

3. *I am often preoccupied with thoughts of food.* (Do you often think about food while performing routine tasks? Are your food thoughts obsessive? Can you go for long periods of time and not think about food?)

4. *I binge at least once a month.* (Food-bingeing is a classic symptom of food addiction. It could involve eating a half gallon of ice cream at one sitting or twenty ice cream bars in four hours. It is comparable to an alcoholic getting drunk or a drug addict getting stoned. Even a once-a-month food binge is significant and indicative of compulsive and self-destructive behavior.)

5. *I prefer to eat alone.* (Food addicts often prefer to eat alone because they are ashamed of their eating habits. They believe that other people will judge them because of how much they eat. Many eat alone in cars on a regular basis and avoid public eating. They find ways to sneak food even at home because they don't want family members to observe, judge or attempt to control them.)

6. *Food has a major calming effect on my emotions.* (How often do you eat to kill your feelings? Most food addicts do this every single day. They use food as

a tranquilizer to dampen, eliminate or change an emotional state.)

7. *I often eat until I am physically uncomfortable.* (Do you know when you have had enough to eat? Can you stop eating when your body tells you it is satisfied? Do you often feel stuffed after eating? Do you know what it is like to finish a meal and feel comfortable, or "light"?)

8. *I often sneak food or eat in secret.* (This is a version of question No. 5 and deserves more attention. Sneaking food and eating in secret are signs we are uncomfortable or ashamed about feeding ourselves. It means the act of nurturing has gotten polluted with deeper emotional issues such as control, perfection, shame and love-deprivation.)

9. *I force myself to eat "normally" in public.* (Do you consciously control or limit the types and amounts of food you eat when other people are present? Do you have concerns that others are eating less than you are eating and does it affect what you choose to eat?)

10. *I often dream about food.* (Dreams come from our unconscious and give important messages about our needs and desires. Dreams that frequently include food are a good indication of how important food has become and usually give an idea about what food symbolizes. Food dreams can indicate addiction and can also point to the powerful underlying issues that drive eating patterns.)

11. *I get anxious when food is not readily available.* (Do you have difficulty tolerating events and situations that do not have food present? Have you become creative in your ability to include food in your daily activities?)

12. *I eat whenever I feel a strong emotion.* (This question is related to question No. 6. How often do you go directly to food when you have an intense emotion? You may consider the emotion negative [anger, anxiety, sadness] or positive [love, lust, joy] but either way you eat.)

Let's assume you answered yes to at least three of the questions and know you have a food addiction. What now? What do you do now?

Here is what *not* to do. Do not go into self-hate or self-condemnation. Resist the temptation to put yourself down because you have discovered a personal flaw. I repeat . . . you are in good company. Many of us are food addicts. Food addiction does not mean we are bad. It means we are part of a large group of people who suffer from the same problem and can join together to help each other.

What to do? The answer is simple—pray!

Here's why pray is your first response: Being addicted to anything, be it food, alcohol or an idea, means you are destructively out-of-control. The addiction is harmful to your well-being and can often be life-threatening. Addiction eliminates choice and freedom and creates helplessness and hopelessness.

Once we are helpless and hopeless, we are at what all twelve-step programs call the "bottom." The bottom is a dark, empty place in which we finally face ourselves and our addiction. We can drop no farther and are unable to go upward on our own power. We have reached what analyst and author Linda Leonard calls "the abyss." It is both the worst and best place we have ever been.

Says Leonard:

*"The journey of the addict takes him inexorably into the abyss of darkness, the depths of despair, where he reaches bottom and asks for help. It is in that long journey into night's despair that he is forced to face his powerlessness."*

*"The first step in any process of recovery is to admit that one is powerless over one's addiction and that one's life has become unmanageable."*

*"These admissions of powerlessness can turn the intense humiliation and helplessness one feels in the abyss to humility and hope. The pivotal point in transforming an addiction is letting go——surrender . . . the abyss is the most significant place for human transformation."*

Dr. Leonard is telling us the abyss is the place in which we truly learn how to pray. It is here that we scream out our need and lose all pretense of being self-sufficient. Here, prayer explodes the boundaries of form, ritual and dogma and assumes an authenticity that is as real as breathing.

Leonard supports her faith in the usefulness of the abyss by quoting Rainer Maria Rilke, possibly the most inspired spiritual poet of the last century.

> *"The strong, inwardly quivering bridge of the Mediator has sense only where the abyss is granted between God and us . . . but this very abyss is full of the darkness of God, and where one experiences it, let him climb down and howl in it (that is more necessary than to cross over it)."*

> *"Only to him for whom the abyss, too, has been a dwelling place do the heavens before him turn about and everything deeply and profoundly of this world that the Church embez-zled for the Beyond, comes back; all the angels decide, singing praises, in favor of earth."*

Rilke is affirming the life-transforming power of the worst thing we can experience in life—the abyss. He asks us to climb into it and howl (pray) and emphasizes this howling is more important than passing through and out of that terrible place. He assures us we are not alone there but are blessed by the "darkness of God," a quality of Divine Presence that is only known by those who endure this strange and dark place of ultimate surrender.

Addiction of any kind is painful. Left unchecked, it will always lead us to our personal abyss. Food addiction, in my opinion, may be the most difficult of all addictions because one cannot abstain from eating. We can eliminate alcohol, cigarettes and drugs from our everyday existence, but we have to eat.

Food must remain part of our daily routine, and we must partake of at least a portion of that substance to which we are addicted. Thus, food addiction may have the most potential to lead us to helplessness and, ultimately, the abyss.

Weight loss can seem so ordinary. It is a regular part of life. But that should not cause us to lose sight of the pain and suffering excess weight can cause.

Many of us find significant and sustained weight loss impossible. We try and try to keep the weight off, but nothing works. We are addicted and we are out of control and we hate ourselves for it.

We feel totally incapable of change, while at the same time knowing change is necessary. We are at the abyss, and we know it. Thank God for prayer.

### The Prayer of the Abyss

The prayer of the abyss is the prayer of the addict. It is truly a howling, an instinctive cry that emerges from the deepest corner of our being. It requires no lessons or lectionaries, no proper names for God and no final amen. It is so powerful that it shatters our resistance to receiving and all our images of God. We are naked in the dark with our Maker, and we have nothing left to say but "Help me."

The prayer of the abyss, the prayer that is cried in utter darkness, may be the most powerfully fertile prayer we ever pray. Darkness is a place we avoid. We always prefer light, but, paradoxically, the best beginnings occur in the darkest environments. No one plants a seed in the sun. A seed needs the black loam of soil. It wants to be hidden from even the slightest glimmer of sunshine until it can send roots even deeper into darkness and grow strong enough to absorb the light to which it aspires.

Every human being is conceived, then nurtured for months in the wet, warm darkness of the mother's womb. We accept this darkness as good and natural even though it is characterized by total helplessness and dependency on the mother. This darkness is welcomed, even enjoyed. It is a necessary part of our life cycle that must not be prematurely interrupted. We are not introduced to light until we have developed the strength to endure it.

The prayer of the abyss is the prayer of the seed in darkness. In this space of no light, our shells crack open and, instead of destruction, we are met with a mysterious nurture that draws us into an expansion and potential that we could never imagine. What acorn can foresee an oak? What tiny rocklike kernel of existence could envision that it would give birth to corn or an apple or an aspen or a redwood?

We always approach the abyss with fear, yet it is the place we learn to pray the most important prayers of our lives. These prayers are seed-prayers. They are broken-open prayers that destroy the rigid self-limiting and God-limiting bonds to which we have grown so attached. Without these prayers we would remain kernel-bound;

small, constricted and completely unaware of the great creative mystery that we are.

Rather than fear the abyss, we could draw courage from Rilke's words and welcome it. Instead of retreating from its perceived horrors, we could reverse our path and climb down into the middle of it and howl our broken-open seed-prayers until our roots emerge and a wondrous green shoot appears and leads us to the light.

I have faith in the fabric of the universe and its Creator. I have faith that all things, all events, all situations and all conditions, however painful and dark, are potential sources of transformation and new life. I have faith that every abyss, with no exception, is actually a womb and that every hardened shell contains the blueprint of a magnificent plant.

I have faith that all darkness is, as Rilke states, "full of the darkness of God." I have faith, like Rumi, that there is no reality but God and there is only God. And, finally, I have faith, like Jesus, that every crucifixion can be followed by a resurrection.

Addiction is an opportunity for faith. We can use it to let go of our restrictive and often dysfunctional beliefs about ourselves and God. We can allow its unrelenting and merciless exposure of our helplessness to teach us about surrender. And in the midst of the darkness of our personal abyss, we can discover the miraculous power of prayer.

The prayer of addiction is the prayer of the abyss and, as such, it cannot be complex or wordy. It is a simple cry that every one of us can make with no preparation or training. It is the cry we all make when we emerge from our mother's body and greet the light for the first time. It is full of helplessness and confusion . . . need and hope. It is so heartfelt and tender that no mother can resist it. It is at once a scream for help and an announcement of a new being. Thank God for that prayer.

> *What if the most intense helplessness and despair you have ever felt was actually a state of grace? What if your addiction was God's way of telling you to let go and surrender to his love? How would you pray then?*

## Ten

# PRAYER AND WEIGHT LOSS—QUESTIONS AND ANSWERS

---

*"Be helpless and dumbfounded,
unable to say yes or no.*

*Then a stretcher will come
from grace to gather us up."*

—Jelaludin Rumi

---

Over the last year, I have received thousands of e-mails asking questions about the Prayer Diet. I have listed and responded to a number of them below. Some questions were asked by dieters and a few, like the first one, were unique but still deserving of a response. Each question seemed to be sincere and significant, therefore I have attempted to give as complete a response as possible.

## Question

*"I thought you were a man of God. Aren't you just doing this Prayer Diet thing as another way to hype the gullible public into paying you big bucks?"*

## Response

I received this question from one brave soul who I am sure is not alone in his cynicism. The issue of spirituality and financial gain is relevant, and if I had not received this question, I would have written it myself.

I began asking it the first day I received 1,000 e-mails in response to my July 17, 2000, eDiets article. I realized something amazing was happening, and I would have been a fool to ignore the financial potential. Immediately, I returned to an internal dialogue I have had for thirty years.

Yes, I am what most would call a man of God. I am an ordained minister and spiritual teacher. I have been practicing my vocation since age fifteen. I believe God has given me certain gifts and expects me to use them. He also expects me to be responsible for the rewards those gifts produce.

When I was younger, my dialogue also included a belief that a man of God was not supposed to be a man of the world. I thought a minister or spiritual teacher should be "above it all." Money and material things were tainted and could even be dangerous distractions from more lofty pursuits.

I was a theological and philosophical dualist who was convinced the material world and the spiritual world were inherently different. I was under the mistaken impression that I could have one without the other, that I should pursue the spiritual and attempt to cleanse myself of the material. This position has a long history in Christian tradition. It is not Biblical, but it has been influential in religious circles. Mine included.

> What if you believed God could use you in his service no matter who you are or even who you've been? What if your imperfections and shortcomings were an essential part of his plan for your life? What, then, would be your prayer?

My theology required that I find an answer to this important question. How can I remain true to my calling and potentially prosper in a material world? Here is my answer.

Both Jewish and Christian traditions teach that God created the material universe. At every step of the process, he looked at what he was doing and pronounced it good. He made stars, planets, oceans, plants, animals and humans—all had material form and all were good. The Christian tradition also teaches that God himself became flesh in the person of Jesus.

I am a product of these traditions and accept these statements as truth. I believe materiality is an essential part of reality and that meaningful spiritual growth can only occur in relationship to it. We were never meant to reject or discount the physicality of God's creation. We were meant to enjoy it!

This means that I am called to live in this material world as a person who is both material and spiritual. I cannot use my spirituality as a convenient way to avoid the harsh realities and incredible joys of the material world. I must find a way to live, as Carl Jung would say, "between the polarities." It is here that I will find the transforming answers to my questions.

On one side of the polarity sits the part of me that wants to be as close to God as possible. On the other side is my capitalist part, which compels me to enjoy every aspect of materiality—such things as good food, nice houses and fast computers. Both parts of me are real and true. Neither can be ignored or avoided.

I have discovered that real growth and personal integrity require that I allow both sides to stay in constant dialogue. Each has a contribution to the other. One without the other becomes unbalanced and potentially dysfunctional. Spirituality without materiality is airy, dry, heartless and out of touch with the wonder of creation.

Materiality without spirituality is cynical, addictive and ultimately violent and self-destructive.

Do I want to prosper financially from this book? Of course. Do I also want this book to be a manifestation of God's purpose in my life and a gift to every person who reads it? Absolutely. In the meantime, I will do my best to continue my inner dialogue and live as responsibly as I can. May God guide my way.

> *What if you believed that God's favorite way of answering prayer was through people? Which of your prayers have already been answered and through whom?*

## Question

*"I prayed the Dieter's Prayer for two weeks. The first week I lost six pounds and the second I lost four pounds. Is this real? Am I fooling myself?"*

## Response

I have received dozens of e-mails almost identical to this one. My answer is always the same. Your scale is not lying to you. Yes, your weight loss is real, and, yes, your prayer is being answered. Keep praying. Don't forget to keep praying.

I am repeating myself because many chronically over-weight people have low self-esteem. This usually includes a resistance to receiving gifts, and weight loss is perceived as a gift. When the gift is larger than we think we deserve, we resist it. What better way to self-sabotage than to stop praying for weight loss as soon as we lose some weight?

I receive regular feedback from prayer dieters, and many of them indicate the tendency to limit what one receives is prevalent. Your task is to keep praying and to let God decide what you deserve. He will be far more generous than you can imagine.

> *What if your image of God is too small? What if God is bigger, wiser, more powerful, more loving and more caring than you could possibly ever imagine? Will you pray for God to open your mind and expand your imagination?*

## Question

*"I have not prayed for years. Is this a problem?"*

Absolutely not. It does not matter when you prayed last. God has been waiting patiently for your call. He is always glad to hear from you. Meister Eckhart would say we may leave God, but God never leaves us. He remains at the door of our hearts waiting, without judgment, for us to indicate even slightly that we are ready for contact. Anything less would be contrary to His nature.

This question is wonderful because it reminds us that we have been on a long and unnecessary trip and need to return to the One who always welcomes us. We need not fear to knock on the door. We only need to open our hearts to the love that embraces us when we reach out our hands.

> *"Come, come, whoever you are! Wanderer,*
> *worshiper, lover of leaving*
>
> *Come, this is not a caravan of despair.*
> *It doesn't matter if you've broken*
> *your vow a thousand times, still*
>
> *Come, and yet again, come!"*
>
> —Rumi

## Question

*"Is being fat bad, or a sin, or a punishment from God?"*

## Response

Americans, like all affluent people, are fat-haters. We think thin is beautiful and fat is ugly. Almost every person who has grown up in our society is infected with this nasty perception. It is shameful and tragic we think this way, but we do.

Given that the majority (55 percent) of us are overweight it is amazing we sustain such a negative attitude about ourselves. One would think we would look around and say, "Hey guys, the majority of us are this way. Why don't we decide it's O.K.?" But that perceptional shift may never come.

In addition to society's negative attitude about weight gain, this question also reflects inaccurate theology. The questioner is assuming God thinks like Americans. If Americans were God, then, of course, being fat would be a sin. We would have our own set of commandments and one of the first would be, "Thou shalt not get fat."

But God remains God and Americans remain as human as ever, contrary to what a few of us may believe. Therefore, the simple answer to the question is: *It is not a sin to be fat, nor is it a punishment.*

Being fat is not a sign of evil and does not mean you are bad. God does not hate you for being overweight. He will not reject you because you are five or twenty-five or 150 pounds heavier than you need to be. He understands the causes of your weight gain and is filled with compassion for your struggle.

No, you are not "bad" if you are overweight. In fact, if you are chronically overweight, it is probably due to something beyond your control. It is a manifestation of an addiction more difficult to manage than drugs or cigarettes.

Too often, many of us would rather think we are bad for being fat. That gives us at least an illusion of control. We think someday we will be "good," will learn self-discipline and will lose those ugly pounds. I suggest we would be better off if we let go of the "bad" idea and faced the real truth. We are not bad. We are addicted.

This knowledge would put us in a position to deal with our weight and ourselves.

Remember, God loves you *and* your body, whatever the condition. He is compassionate and understanding and wants to help you grow and heal and prosper. He does not want you to hate yourself for being fat. Trust that, and you will find more useful and transforming interpretations of your weight will appear.

> What if your excess weight is God's way of answering one of your most important prayers? Which one would it be?

## Question

*"I want to pray for weight loss, but I am not sure I deserve God's help with this. What can I do?"*

## Response

The first thing you can do is realize you are not alone. Many of us feel this way. We think we have to be "good" before God will help us. The problem is not with God but our own thinking. We are the ones who believe we are not deserving of his love, protection or support, and we project this attitude onto God. Then we are afraid to ask for his help.

Too often, we confuse our own personal psychology with theology. If we have a lot of self-judgment, we imagine God feels the same way about us. It is important to realize that God loves us more than we love ourselves.

God does not think you are undeserving of his help or forgiveness. He wants you to ask him for support, and your weight is a good place to start.

This question is important because it may affect every aspect of your prayer life. If you feel undeserving, you may stop yourself from asking God to help you and that would be a tragedy.

I remember a story someone told me about a woman who died and went to heaven. When she arrived, she met St. Peter, who told her he would start by giving her a tour.

He walked her through a magnificent mansion full of breathtaking rooms until they finally stopped in front of a massive door. St. Peter told her this door led to the saddest room in heaven. When the door opened, the woman saw an enormous space full of beautifully wrapped presents.

It was such a lovely sight she could not imagine why it was called the saddest room. St. Peter responded, "my dear, these are all the gifts that God has offered His children on earth that have not been accepted. Each recipient has refused them because they were sure they were undeserving."

We have all refused gifts from God because we thought we did not deserve them. The ability to lose weight is only one of them. I advise you to pray for weight loss without hesitation. Pray for anything else you want.

Then, open your heart, mind and body to receive the wonderful gifts God wants to shower upon you. Soon

you will find the idea of deserving was irrelevant and enjoying the gifts is what it's all about.

## Question

*"Is prayer all I need to lose weight?"*
*Yes and No.*

## Response

Yes, prayer is all you need to lose weight. More
specifically, a constant-prayer diet is all you need. What is
a constant-prayer diet? A constant-prayer diet that creates and sustains meaningful weight loss must have a
number of ingredients. Here are the basics.

### THE CONSTANT-PRAYER DIET

1. *You must pray constantly.* Prayer must become a way
   of life. You must learn to pray through everything
   you do, all the time. Prayer has to be as important
   as breathing.

   This may seem difficult, but it is not. Praying the
   Dieter's Prayer is a great beginning to making
   prayer an intimate constant in your daily life.
   Praying the additional prayers I have recommended
   will support this practice. Experiencing the wonderful answers that are the results of prayer will
   also increase your desire and commitment.
2. *You must open yourself to God's answers to your prayer.*

The Prayer for Openness and Vision will help you with this task. You need to continually develop your ability to see God's specific answers to your requests for guidance and healing. Blindness due to prejudice and ignorance will prevent you from receiving his best gifts.

3. *Once you become aware of God's guidance, you must follow it to the best of your ability*. I am reminded of a story Caroline Myss (a medical intuitive and spiritual teacher) told in one of her speeches. A single woman asked her if God would help her find that special man she so dearly wanted. Caroline said, "Yes, God will help you, but he might ask you to move to West Virginia first. Would you go?" The questioner had great difficulty saying yes.

Prayer requires response, both from God and from the person who prays. We cannot expect to pray, then lose weight without responsibility. Our prayer invites God to participate in our lives. When that happens, things change and events occur we could never predict. Yes, you can rely on prayer only for weight loss and it will bring far more than a lower pants size.

Now for the "no" answer . . . Prayer alone is not enough to sustain weight loss. Most of us are not going to make prayer a way of life. We won't become totally committed to prayer. If that is the case and we still want to pray, what can we do?

Picture a bicycle wheel. The hub is in the center and

spokes radiate evenly out to the rim, which supports the tire. If each part does its job, the wheel rolls easily and the bike works perfectly.

Now imagine the wheel representing your weight-loss process. If each part functions properly, you will lose weight and keep it off. Now substitute prayer for the hub. It is at the center of the wheel and is necessary to the effective function of all the other parts. But it is not the only part that's important. The spokes, the rim and the tire all play their role in the creation and "healthy" function of the wheel . . . or weight-loss process.

Using this analogy, we can see prayer is essential and central but does not stand alone. Other ingredients are necessary for the process to work. Each has its particular function but is influenced by the center, or prayer. Those other parts are specific and identifiable, and I would like to briefly mention them. Each should be infused and guided by prayer.

### Factors That Support Prayer and Weight Loss

1. We must learn to heal and manage our difficult emotions. This requires the wise and persistent use of psychology and in-depth inner work. I cannot overemphasize this point. No one ever truly manages weight problems without confronting and healing inner pain and trauma. I have never met an exception to this rule. We must learn what we are "eating to kill" and must find healthy means of satisfying our deeper needs and desires.

2. We must build a strong base of self-esteem and self-love. Weight loss is a manifestation of self-care. We cannot lose weight and keep it off if we do not like ourselves. While losing weight can be a factor in increased self-esteem, it will not be enough by itself. We must learn attitudes and behaviors that nurture our sense of value, worthiness and self-image.

3. We must learn to eat consciously. As I mentioned earlier, most overweight individuals become unconscious when they eat. This means they eat with no awareness of taste, satisfaction or amount. If we want to lose weight and sustain that weight loss, we must learn to be fully alert every time we encounter food.

Prayer can become our central support for the three important functions above. It can lead us to the right psychological guides (books, workshops, counselors, etc.), open us to their wisdom and guidance and give us the courage to confront the issues that emerge from that relationship.

Prayer can also help us locate and attain thoughts and behaviors that support our increasing self-esteem and self-love. It reminds us our Creator made us and we are all creatures of beauty and priceless value in His eyes.

Finally, prayer can be a technique for increasing consciousness. For many prayer dieters, praying just before eating makes them intensely aware of food and their relationship with it.

Whether you prefer my yes or no answer, I hope you will see that prayer can be an essential factor in your weight-loss process. Initially, you may not know the power of prayer, so I ask you to begin praying as much as you can, to stay open to the answers you receive and then to follow God's guidance.

## Question

*"Is prayer more effective than willpower?"*

## Response

Any veteran of the battles of weight loss knows will-power is grossly overrated. It is only effective for the short term and is never strong enough to overcome the enormous energies that drive us to overeat. Many a dieter has used willpower to lose five, ten or twenty-five pounds only to be defeated and disillusioned.

I have listened to individuals who have no weight issues comment about an overweight person's apparent lack of willpower and self-discipline. They mistakenly assume that a simple decision to eat less, plus a little exercise, will solve the problem.

On occasion, I ask these self-appointed weight gurus if there is any aspect of their lives they cannot control. Most often they answer no. From that moment there is no room for communication, and I quickly change the subject.

I recently attended a friend's wedding. When it was

time for the wedding dinner, I found the first empty chair and sat down. I began a conversation with a man, and we discussed the weather, politics and numerous other subjects. Finally, he asked what I did for a living, and I told him I wrote for an Internet diet service.

As soon as he heard the words "diet" and "weight loss," he launched into a biased and judgmental sermonette about the "problem with overweight people." He said he had no compassion for overweight persons because they were obviously unwilling to control their eating. He felt weight was simply a matter of self-discipline and that all overweight people just needed to face that fact and get on with it.

I listened for a few moments, then asked him if there was any aspect of his life that was out of his control. No, he responded. I then asked if he realized that his rather severe judgments about obese people was an example of being out of control.

He looked at me as if I was an idiot, and the conversation came to a screeching halt. I finished my meal and left the party. I don't think I will ever see this person again, but I am sure I will encounter that same ignorant attitude about weight loss and willpower.

The fact of the matter is willpower is not comparable to prayer. Willpower is momentary; it was never designed to sustain us for the long term. Prayer, however, gives us access to infinite energy that, by definition, has no limit. When we pray, we connect to a source that is both within and around us. It sustains us, supports us, fills us and goes before us. Unlike willpower, that source does not base its care and nurture on hope or hype, excitement or desperation. It is there rain or shine, day or night, constantly encouraging us and leading us to our goal.

I have learned by trial and many errors, to substitute prayer for willpower, especially when it comes to weight loss. I would much rather rely on divine power than my own.

### Question

*"Can I pray for other people to lose weight?"*

### Response

Of course you can. People pray for others every moment of every day with miraculous results. I always pray for everyone on the Prayer Diet and encourage and accept the prayers of others.

I often suggest prayer dieters form informal prayer groups to pray for each other and people outside their group. Praying for others seems to increase our ability to pray and receive guidance. It also helps everyone lose weight.

There is a second question that often comes with this one.

## Question

*"Can I pray for someone to lose weight without telling them?"*

## Response

Yes, you can. Sometimes it is even best that you pray in secret. Not everyone is thrilled to be told they are on your weight-loss prayer list. I am, of course, but I accept every prayer I can get. You might call me spiritually greedy, but I prefer to call it needy.

Yes, pray for anyone you like. God will use your prayer for their best interest. They need never know.

## Question

*"My spouse does not believe in the power of prayer. What should I do?"*

Very few of us live with family members who are spiritually identical. There are always differences, sometimes great, sometimes small. You may, however, be married to someone who thinks the Prayer Diet is absurd. That poses a problem, but not one that is insurmountable.

If your spouse thinks prayer is silly, or that praying for weight loss is useless, I recommend you take the path of least resistance. Pray in secret. Do not make prayer a point of conflict. Simply pray in private. God will hear you and understand. Besides, nothing will prove your point better than significant weight loss.

Having a spouse who does not believe in prayer does not mean you married the wrong person. Neither does it mean you must work hard to change their mind. After almost thirty years of working with couples with similar difficulties, I believe differences are there for a reason. Our task is not to make our spouse wrong but to explore the deeper reason for the differences.

When problems arise in marriages, the easiest thing to do is blame your partner. You may be perfectly correct in your description of your partner's guilt, but you will not be one step closer to a solution. In fact, being right is the best way to end up divorced. There is a line in *A Course In Miracles* that says the following:

*"Would you rather be right or happy?"*

If you want to make real progress in your marriage when problems appear, you need to ask yourself this question over and over. Then pray for guidance and open yourself to an answer you have never considered. It will come.

### Question

*"I was sexually abused as a child, and I am sure it has contributed to my weight problem. Can I pray to have my past healed?*

## Response

Of course you can pray for the healing of your past and especially for this very painful issue. You are correct that it is related to weight gain. Many overweight people report childhood sexual abuse and have often discovered it affects lifelong eating patterns. Given the pain and trauma associated with this issue, I would like to give some more advice.

Most people who have been abused would rather not remember it. This is a natural reaction to a humiliating and often devastating experience. It would also be understandable if the abused individual wanted to use prayer to wipe the trauma from her or his memory. Why hold on to a horrible event if prayer could make it disappear?

Understand that *prayer is not a religious substitute for denial*. If you attempt to use prayer as a tool of avoidance, you will be ignoring the inner work that is necessary for healing. In addition, you may miss the lessons God has implanted in the recovery process.

Life is far more complex than it seems, and God is even more mysterious. Painful events contain great meaning. The discovery of that meaning can transform our lives more significantly than the original event harmed us. This process takes courage and a lot of faith, but it is well worth the effort.

You can and should pray for God to heal the pain and trauma of your past. You need and deserve it. At the same time, you would do well to ask God to help you see and learn the lessons embedded in your recovery process. You may come to realize that God can use any life crisis to your advantage.

## Question

*"I want to try the Prayer Diet, but I think I would do better with support. Is it O.K. to start a prayer group that focuses only on weight loss?"*

Yes, it is more than O.K. It is a great idea. Most of us do much better at everything if we have a support group to encourage us. I suggest you begin praying for the right people to show up and start the group as soon as possible. Here is a suggested meeting structure.

1. Each group meeting has a moderator who leads the group through each step. The moderator changes every week. Meeting once a week is usually best.
2. Start by praying the Dieter's Prayer aloud as a group.
3. Each member shares their experience with the Dieter's Prayer over the last week. Anyone who didn't pray the prayer is not judged but is encouraged to start again.

   In addition to weight loss, each participant should share additional experiences caused by the prayer. These include increased awareness of eating patterns and food, changing relationships and effects on self-esteem and self-image.
4. Pray aloud and discuss the significance of the other

four prayers described in Chapter 5, Maintaining Weight Loss. These prayers and the material they generate are as important as the Dieter's Prayer.

5. Conclude the meeting by holding hands and praying spontaneously.

## Question

*"Do the members of my Prayer Diet group have to hold my religious beliefs?"*

## Response

No, group members do not have to have the same religious beliefs. This means your group could include Baptists, Methodists, Catholics, Jews, Hindus, Muslims, New Agers and agnostics. In my experience, the more diverse the group, the better.

The only requirement is that everyone must agree that differences are acceptable. Ultimately, the only rule for a Prayer Diet group is that everyone agrees to pray.

*"Throughout this book you have used different titles for God. Why do you do that?"*

Actually, I would prefer to drop all names and titles for God. First because I feel so intimately connected that a title has a distancing effect. Second because God is essentially a mystery and ineffable. He/She/It is beyond my ability to name and therefore limit. When I do have to use a title for God, I always feel a bit awkward but I choose the name or title that is most comfortable for my audience.

I have used titles for God in this book based solely on prayerful intuition. However, I firmly believe that you should use titles and names that are comfortable for you. I have no problem with any God-name changes you want to make in any of the prayers I have written.

Given that God is not neurotic, I assume that She does not require a specific name in order to respond to your prayers. He listens to your heart and not your words, as Rumi has so eloquently reminded us.

## Question

*"I am not comfortable with some of the wording in the Dieter's Prayer. Can I change it, and will that change the results?"*

I wrote the Dieter's Prayer, and it is not sacred or sacrosanct. Neither is it a magic formula. Of course you can change it, and I am sure God will still respond with care and love.

I had one reservation about changing the prayer, but as I began to write it down, I realized that letting go and trusting you and your relationship with God is far wiser than attempting to control or direct you. I will conclude my answer with a wonderful quote from St. Augustine:

*"Love God and do what you will."*

## Question

*"When I pray and ask God to help me, I feel as if I am losing control of my life. This is very hard for me. What can I do about this?"*

First, recognize you are not alone. Asking for help is hard for most of us, especially those who need to feel in charge and in control of just about everything. Praying for God's help is an admission we are not able to control some aspect of our lives and often have great resistance to it. In addition, prayer requires us to do something that may seem impossible to us control freaks—"Let go and let God."

Prayer takes matters out of our hands and puts them into the hands of our Divine Source. It always activates any and all of our "control issues." I have chosen a phrase often used by therapists because it goes to the heart of this rather difficult psychological process.

A control issue is a complex of needs, wants and fears that involves our natural struggle to grow beyond dependency and become an independent, self-sufficient individual.

If that process is hindered or blocked by dysfunctional parenting, we may find ourselves obsessed with a desire to control each and every aspect of our lives. Then we often interpret any suggestion to "let go" as a threat to our well-being.

Most of us have some degree of control issues, and prayer pushes them into our emotional faces. I remember a fifty-year-old client who once said,

> *"Matthew, this prayer thing is so hard for me. Every time I start to pray, I become anxious. I feel like I am giving up control of my life, and I have worked for thirty years to take charge of everything that was important to me. I really want to lose weight, and it is clear that I can't do it alone. But I really want to do it myself. I hate asking for help, and I hate feeling weak and helpless. In addition, I am afraid God will not be there to catch me when I step into that abyss."*

This man spoke for millions of us. Control is important, and praying makes us feel out of control. No wonder we resist it. But there is some good news in the midst of this control struggle. Being out of control is where we need to be.

Being out of control means we are finally ready to be helped, healed and guided. Our control needs have blinded us to the very help we earnestly seek. Being out of control does not put us in the terrible chaos we fear will kill us. It opens us to receive God's blessing and love. Remember the excerpt from Rumi: *"Be helpless and dumbfounded, unable to say yes or no. Then a stretcher will come from grace and gather us up."*

Rumi understands the power of our need to control. He also understands the importance of learning to let go. He is encouraging us to do the exact opposite of what we usually attempt (control) and he assures us it is in our helplessness that God will act. Grace will come with a stretcher and take us wherever we need to go.

I remember the first time I read this poem. I began to cry with relief. I felt the iron cable of control that had bound and restricted me for so long break and drop away. I knew I was helpless. I knew I was dumbfounded. I knew I could not "make" anything happen in my life. I knew I needed a stretcher, and I absolutely knew I needed grace. I still cry every time I read these healing words. Thank God this whole thing is not up to me. Thank God for grace and for always running down the road to meet me. Thank God for making prayer and giving me such a natural vehicle for letting go.

### Question

*"You have suggested that we pray for the healing of our food addiction. Can we pray the same prayers for drug and alcohol addiction?"*

### Response

Of course. The substance (such as food, alcohol or drugs) is far less important than the addiction itself. You may want to change a few words in the prayers to make them appropriate to the addiction, but the essence is the same.

Prayer, especially the prayer of the abyss, makes an enormous difference in recovery from addiction. If you have an addiction of any kind, you would be wise to pray every day about everything that confronts you. Acquiring this habit will assure you of consistent and miraculous support for your recovery.

## Question

*"What if I pray and I don't lose weight?"*

This question is important because it is real. Sometimes we pray for weight loss and we don't lose a pound. What does it mean? Does it mean that prayer is useless? Does it mean we are doing something wrong? Does it mean God doesn't care? I have the same answer to all three questions—no, no, no. Prayer works. You have not done something wrong, and God does care about you and your weight problem. Why, then, are you not losing weight?

Over my lifetime, I have prayed thousands of prayers asking for very specific results. I have often gotten answers that were different from my requests. On occasion, I have felt disappointed about this apparent disrespect for my needs and desires. But I have learned to look at my prayer results with a more trusting eye, and that has made all the difference.

If you pray for weight loss and don't lose weight, you could use that experience to decide prayer is useless or that God doesn't care. I recommend a different perspective. Assume the prayer *is* being answered, and you have yet to realize its form. This perspective requires faith and trust in God's wisdom. It also requires us to let go of our attachment to a specific outcome . . . weight loss . . . and open ourselves to a greater possibility. I would like to share an example from my own life.

In 1980, my wife and I left a successful counseling practice in Boston and moved to Los Angeles. We expected to quickly repeat what we had created on the East Coast and looked forward to plenty of clients and lots of money.

Every day I prayed for God's blessing on our new practice. Every day I asked God's to help us prosper. Every day we spent money on advertising, rent, food and other bills. And every day nothing happened. In five short months we spent every cent we had. Before we knew what was happening, we were broke.

We were humiliated, frightened, confused and lost. But we were not abandoned. My prayers for prosperity were being answered in a fashion that I could not understand. We were being directed to leave L.A. We were being led to another place and other lessons. Within a year, we were settled in San Diego with new friends and a blossoming practice. My prayers were answered through a process and form that I could never have imagined.

If you have prayed diligently for weight loss and you have not lost a single ounce, there is only one thing to do. Keep praying and open yourself to the possibility that God has something even more wonderful in store for you. Eventually you may lose weight, but something else must occur. Relax and continue praying.

## Question

*"Can I pray even if I am not sure that God exists?"*

## Response

Julia Cameron, in her wonderful book, *The Artist's Way,* has a provocative answer to this question.

> *"It's my experience that we're much more afraid that there might be a God than we are that there might not be . . . People talk about how dreadful it would be if there were no God. I think such talk is hooey. Most of us are a lot more comfortable feeling we're not being watched too closely.*
>
> *If there is a responsive creative force that does hear us and act on our behalf, then we may really be able to do some things. The jig, in short, is up: God knows that the sky's the limit."*

Yes, you can pray even if you are not sure there is a God. Pray and expect an answer. When you begin to lose weight you might just decide this God thing is a good idea and God knows what you will pray for next. Remember, the only thing that stands between you and a life-changing experience of God is your ambivalence. For just a moment, let go and ask for help. Or just let go. Nothing else is necessary.

*What if God always answers your prayer with a wisdom greater than your own? What if the gifts he wants to give you are bigger and more magnificent than those you have requested? How, then, would you pray?*

## Eleven

# CONTINUING THE JOURNEY

———————— ∞ ————————

*"So the sea journey goes on, and who knows where!*
*Just to be held by the ocean is the best luck*
*we could have. It's a total waking-up!*

*Why should we grieve that we've been sleeping?*
*It doesn't matter how long we have been unconscious.*

*We're groggy, but let the guilt go.*
*Feel the motions of tenderness*
*around you, the buoyancy."*

—Jelaludin Rumi

———————— ∞ ————————

With all its power, prayer is not a magic bullet that will forever eliminate the monster of weight gain. We cannot pray once and then eat what we will. We must learn to pray more and more until it becomes as frequent as our need for food. The desire to eat, whether motivated by natural hunger or unnatural compulsion, will be an invitation to pray.

If we are to achieve and maintain weight loss, we must view it as a journey, not a destination. Proper care of our body is an ongoing process, not a completed fact. From my point of view, this is good news, not bad. It means we can learn and grow every day from our attention to the needs of our physical selves and from the spiritual growth it engenders.

I have included the following guidelines as additional support for your journey. Each item and attitude has been useful and often crucial to my own process of weight loss and spiritual growth. I hope you will find them as helpful and healing as I have.

## Guidelines for Your Continued Journey

1. *Expect to be surprised.* Prayer is a natural and ordinary expression of our humanity, and it is designed to introduce us to the mystery of life and God. Constant prayer will create events, attitudes and circumstances you cannot predict. It will bring weight loss, but it will also open your heart and mind to a new vision of what it means to be you.

2. *Don't spend time with discouragers*. We all need encouragement for our prayer and weight-loss journey. You will do better if you avoid constant contact with individuals who do not support your goals and practices. Making conscious choices about relationships that nurture us is a sign of positive growth. Don't allow your friends or family to block your progress.

   This guideline is difficult for many people because they feel guilty or disloyal avoiding individuals they have been close to. So remember what your priorities are and what effect these people have on your growth and healing.

   Alcoholics cannot hang out with persons who constantly offer them a drink. You cannot afford to spend time with individuals who discourage you from prayer or weight loss. This is the time to care for yourself and to protect yourself from unnecessary difficulties. Do what you have to do. In the end, you will be happy you did.

3. *Pray whether you feel like it or not*. Sometimes you will want to pray, and sometimes you won't. Do it anyway. Eventually your praying will become as natural and easy as breathing and will not be related to how you feel.

   One of the greatest blocks to learning new behavior is allowing a feeling to dictate behavior. The best way to make progress is to pray, and that means doing what the commercial says . . . "Just do it."

You will find feelings change as you pray. So it doesn't matter what you are feeling when you begin. You will usually feel better once you have begun to pray.

4. *Don't stop praying when you have lost all your weight.* This is the time to be most careful. Reaching a weight-loss goal is wonderful, and we can become so excited about the accomplishment that we actually begin to neglect the process that caused it. Remember that weight loss, like spiritual growth, is an ongoing process. Keep praying and be open to new and even more wonderful developments.

   If you continue to pray after you have lost all your weight, you will enter an entirely new phase of spiritual growth. You will discover that praying for weight loss was preliminary to the real and miraculous power of prayer. Trust me, it's worth it.

5. *Find other people to pray with.* Praying alone is fine, and praying with others is even better. Weight-loss prayer groups and prayer partners are superb sources of comfort, support and encouragement. Tell others what you are doing and invite them to join you. You will be amazed when the "perfect" people show up and give you exactly the care and attention you need.

   I realize this guideline may sound a bit strange, but it is true. I have often been amazed when I prayed and the prayer was answered by the appearance of the most "perfect" person I could have imagined. Your weight-loss prayer group will be filled with these people. I guarantee it.

6. *Allow God to be mysterious*. Prayer connects us to God. God, by definition, is mysterious. His way of attending to your needs may not be according to your limited vision. Expect him to appear in your life in both ordinary and extraordinary ways. Your rigid expectations can be the greatest block to his answers to your prayer. Let go and let God be God. Relax and enjoy the ride.

7. *Practice powerlessness*. Remember that God is in charge and you only need to surrender to his guidance and will. Addiction always returns when we attempt to regain control of our lives and shut God out of the equation. You do not have to fear being powerless. Instead, celebrate it and watch God work in your body and your life.

8. *Learn to enjoy your body*. You have one body in this life. As an old mentor of mine used to say, "Play the cards you are dealt; don't whine about the ones you didn't get." If you use this statement as a guide for caring about your body, you will be much happier. Whatever size or shape you are will not matter if you practice body love.

If enjoying and loving your body is difficult then I suggest you pray often for release from these judgments. Ask God to open your heart to your body. Ask him to teach you how to see your body as a friend and constant companion. Ask for body acceptance and tolerance. Then go ahead and live in your body as fully as you can. God will help you, and your body will love you for it.

9. *Open your heart to love.* We all want to be loved. It is a natural desire. But most of us have a very difficult time receiving it. Our psychological wounds and traumas deter our openness. But, there is good news. We can all learn to be better receivers of love.

   It is no accident that many Scriptures say God is love. If this is accurate, then the following is true: God is love and God is All, so, therefore, All is love. This means love is all around and in you all the time. You must expend little effort to receive love because it is already there. All you have to do is ask God (pray) to open your awareness to it. It will be like opening your eyes in a room that is already filled with light. It was always there, and so were you.

10. *Let go of judgment and pray for compassion.* I remember reading a wonderful statement by Matthew Fox in which he said compassion was the greatest force in the universe. Who can argue with that? I would go even further than that. I believe the ability to see people, situations and especially excess weight through the eyes of compassion is the same as seeing through the eyes of God.

   I believe a compassionate view of reality is the only accurate view, and that is the way God looks at his world. Until you and I can see someone through the eyes of compassion, we cannot see at all.

Judgment clouds vision, and compassion clears it. Judgment is selective and arbitrarily discriminating. It sees one aspect and ignores others. The eyes of judgment are always partially blind. Compassion, on the other hand, embraces all that we are without leaving anything out. Compassion allows us to see past the prejudicial vision of judgment and always leads us to love.

Very little could be more useful and transforming to our lives than compassion. Therefore, it always makes sense to pray for all the compassion we can get and give.

11. *Help someone learn to pray.* To share a thing is to grow that thing in yourself. Sharing prayer is one of the best ways to increase its meaningfulness and power. Every time you speak to a friend or family member about prayer, you will increase your own capacity to pray. In addition, you will be making a contribution to another spiritual traveler.

Remember, you do not have to be an expert on prayer in order to help someone else. You simply have to be honest and share your experience. Tell the other person what prayer has done for you. Tell them how and what you pray, then let God do the rest.

12. *Expect more surprises.* I have offered this guideline

twice because it is so important. I am convinced the main block to our experience of God's power and his constant answers to our prayers is our resistance to surprise. We all become so quickly attached to our expectations and prejudices, we often miss the wonder that God has placed right in front of us. The truth is God's joy is breaking out all around us. If we pray to have our hearts and minds opened to surprises, we will suddenly wake up to the magnificent dance that is life itself. What could be more wonderful?

I could write a thousand more guidelines, but you don't need them. You have prayer. You have all the access you need to the greatest Guide there is. You only need to breathe a prayer, and when you breathe again, you will be filled with its answer. Pray and breathe out. Breathe in and receive the answer.

Guidance is only as far away as your breath. God is even closer. Go and be with both.

> *What if all the guidance you ever needed was as close to you as your breath? How would you breathe? What if you took the deepest breath you could take?*

# ADDENDUM
# LONGER-TERM PRAYER
# AND WEIGHT-LOSS
# RESULTS

In the months since the beginning of the weight-loss prayer project, I have received many more e-mails from individuals who have continued to pray past the initial two-week limit. I have included a sample of some of those e-mails. They continue to confirm the amazing power of prayer and the special commitments of those who pray.

*"Dear Doc, I have been praying the prayer for two months and guess what? I have lost seventeen pounds!!! Can you believe it? I will continue to pray until I lose the other eighty-five I need to shed. I will be in touch."*

*"Dear prayer partner. I have prayed for six weeks and lost ten pounds so far. I am very happy about the weight, but I am even more happy about my spiritual growth. I feel closer to God than I have ever felt in my entire forty-two years of life. Thank you and thank God."*

*"Hi, Doctor Matthew. I must confess that I did not believe that this prayer thing would work, but I tried it because I was desperate. I had tried a million diets, and I failed at every one of them. Praying for God's help has made something happen inside me that I cannot explain. I don't feel so alone anymore. Every time I eat and pray, I feel a presence with me. I feel loved, and I am eating less every day. I have been doing this for about nine weeks and have lost nineteen pounds. Why I didn't pray before I don't know, but I am doing it now and that's all that matters. I am also praying for everyone else who is trying this."*

*"Wow, wow, wow. Prayer is great! I lost weight during the first two-week period (five pounds) and so I decided to go ahead and keep praying. I have done this for four months now. I have lost twenty pounds I plan to pray more and lose more. Thanks so much."*

*"Hello, Matthew. I am one of the prayer people who has been praying to lose weight. I always believed in prayer, and I have many stories about the power of prayer in my life and my family's life. I want you to know that I never thought about praying for weight loss and I am embarrassed to admit it. I know that God cares about my body. I guess I was the one who did not care. Well, I care now, and I have prayed for seven weeks and it works. I have lost fifteen lbs. I have also grown more spiritually in that time than I ever imagined I could. God bless you. You are in my prayers."*

The list grows every day. I am especially excited about the benefits that go beyond weight loss. Many long-term participants report significant spiritual growth, which is equally as important as the weight loss. I had assumed this would be the case, but I am thrilled to see it is actually true. If you are a long-term weight-loss devotee, please contact me and share the results. The contact information is at the end of the book.

# Bibliography

Anderson, Matthew. *Coyote Wisdom—The Prayer Diet.* EDiets.com archived articles.

Barks, Coleman. *Like This: Rumi. 43 Odes.* Athens, GA: Maypop Books, 1990.

Barks, Coleman, trans. *Feeling the Shoulder of the Lion: Poetry and Teaching Stories of Rumi.* Putney, VT: Threshold Books, 1991.

Barks, Coleman, trans. *The Illuminated Rumi: Translations by Coleman Barks.* Illuminations by Michael Green. New York. Broadway Books, 1997.

Barks, Coleman, *Delicious Laughter: Rambunctious Teaching Stories from the Mathnawi Rumi.* Athens, GA: Maypop Books, 1990.

Barks, Coleman and John Moyne, trans. *This Longing: Poetry, Teaching Stories and Letters of Rumi.* Brattleboro, VT: Threshold Books, 1988.

Barks, Coleman. New Rumi translations of *Rumi: We Are Three.* Athens, GA: Maypop Books, 1998.

Cameron, Julia. *The Artist's Way: A Spiritual Path to Higher Creativity.* Los Angeles, CA: Jeremy P. Tarcher/ Perigee, 1992.

# Bibliography

Chopra, Deepak, M. D. *How To Know God: The Soul's Journey into the Mystery of Mysteries*. New York: Harmony Books/ NewYork, 2001.

Dossey, Larry, M. D. *Healing Words: The Power of Prayer and the Practice of Medicine*. San Francisco: Harper SanFrancisco, 1997.

Foundation for Inner Peace. *A Course In Miracles*. New York: Foundation for Inner Peace, 1976.

Fox, Matthew, ed. *Breakthrough: Meister Eckhart's Creation Spirituality in New Translation*. Introduction and commentaries by Matthew Fox. Garden City, New York: Image Books. A Division of Doubleday & Company, Inc., 1980.

Fox, Matthew. *Original Blessing: A Primer in Creation Spirituality*. Santa Fe, New Mexico: Bear and Company.

Grof, Stanislav. *The Adventure of Self-Discovery: Dimensions of Consciousness and New Perspectives in Psychotherapy and Inner Exploration*. State University of New York Press, 1988.

Ladinsky, Daniel, trans. *The Gift: Poems by Hafiz, The Great Sufi Master*. New York: Penguin Compass, 1999.

Leonard, Linda Schierse. *Witness to the Fire: Creativity and the Veil of Addiction*. Boston, MA: Shambala, 1989.

Meier, C.A. *Soul and Body: Essays on the Theories of C. G. Jung*. Santa Monica, San Francisco: The Lapis Press, 1986.

Moyne, John and Coleman Barks, trans. *Say I Am You: Poetry Interspersed with Stories of Rumi and Shams*. Athens, GA: Maypop Books, 1994.

Moyne, John and Coleman Barks, trans. *Open Secret:*

# Bibliography

*Versions of Rumi by John Moyne and Coleman Barks.* Putney, Vermont: Threshold Books, 1984.

Reps, Paul, comp. *Zen Flesh, Zen Bones: A Collection of Zen and Pre-Zen Writings.* Anchor Books. Garden City, New York: Doubleday & Company, Inc., 1976.

Star, Jonathan. *Two Suns Rising: A Collection of Sacred Writings.* New York. Bantam Books, 1997.

Whyte, David. *The House of Belonging: Poems by David Whyte.* Langley, WA: Many Rivers Press, 1997.

Wilber, Ken. *The Eye of the Spirit: An Integral Vision for a World Gone Slightly Mad.* Boston and London: Shambala, 1997.

Woodman, Marion. *Addiction to Perfection: The Still Unravished Bride.* Toronto: Inner City Books, 1982.

# Index

# Index

# Index

## MATTHEW ANDERSON, D. MIN.

For more information about Dr. Anderson's

- Workshops
- Books
- Seminars and Presentations
- Audiotapes
- Individual Consultation by telephone or in person
- Groups
- Articles on the Internet
- Organizational Development Consultation

Call or write to the following:

Telephone—(561) 362–4049 Fax—(561) 362–9041
E-mail—*Mattcoyote@aol.com*

Visit our Web site at *www.Mattcoyote.com*

Matthew Anderson and Associates, Inc.
398 W. Camino Gardens Blvd.
Suite 209
Boca Raton, Florida 33432